The Sensual Slimmer

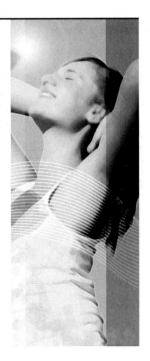

Three Happy Habits for
Successful Weight Loss,
Eating and Quality of Life

DIARMUID LAVELLE

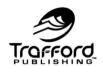
Trafford
PUBLISHING

Order this book online at www.trafford.com/07-2610
or email orders@trafford.com

Most Trafford titles are also available at major online book retailers.

Printed in Victoria, BC, Canada.

ISBN: 978-1-4251-5794-4

We at Trafford believe that it is the responsibility of us all, as both individuals and corporations, to make choices that are environmentally and socially sound. You, in turn, are supporting this responsible conduct each time you purchase a Trafford book, or make use of our publishing services. To find out how you are helping, please visit www.trafford.com/responsiblepublishing.html

Our mission is to efficiently provide the world's finest, most comprehensive book publishing service, enabling every author to experience success. To find out how to publish your book, your way, and have it available worldwide, visit us online at www.trafford.com/10510

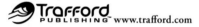 **Trafford** PUBLISHING™ www.trafford.com

North America & international
toll-free: 1 888 232 4444 (USA & Canada)
phone: 250 383 6864 ♦ fax: 250 383 6804 ♦ email: info@trafford.com

The United Kingdom & Europe
phone: +44 (0)1865 722 113 ♦ local rate: 0845 230 9601
facsimile: +44 (0)1865 722 868 ♦ email: info.uk@trafford.com

10 9 8 7 6 5 4 3

Unless otherwise attributed, epigraphs in this book are by the author.

We are how *we eat.*

Contents

Acknowledgments

To my wife Naomi.

To my children Maeve, Caer and Culann.

To my parents Sean and Frances.

To my brothers and sisters, their partners and my nieces and nephews: Sean, Linda, Sean Og, Nuala and Kiaran; Conla, Anne, Maeve and Cathal; Eimer, Eileen and Nuala; Malachy, Kathy, Ross, Dara and Aoife; Frances, Brendan, Siobhan, Niamh, Clara and Siofra. To Maria.

Thanks to my many mentors and supporters. To Anne Breanach who gave me the inspiration for this book; Sean Collins, Rhoda Draper, David Shephard, John Mc Whirter, Kate, Christo and Joseph Scallon; Bill O Hanlon. John Rogers, Ronan, and all the Aikido people. To all my friends: the surfers, mountaineers, drinkers, dreamers, thinkers, lovers, magicians, warriors and rogues. To my lecturers and mentors in archaeology, psychology and philosophy at NUIG. To my teachers in the Presentation, Tailorshill, St. Enda's, Mary's and Castleknock. To the lads in Greenfields. To Paul and Sandra, Joe and Margaret, Ernest and Mary, Hubert and Marie, Pete, Jane, Sean, Bernie and Padraic, Paudie and Kathleen. To Rob, Larissa, Jackie, Richard. To Roseanne, Brian and Mary Avril, Tony, Liz and David, Hugh and

Orla, Alison, James and Maria, Paul, Roy and Margo, William, Ruth and Sean, Bob and Fran. To Maura, Paul, Pat, Adrian, Stephan, Bertrand, Rosemary, Liz and Tommy, Clara and Sharon. To Bernie and Teresa, Freedmar, Lenin, Barbara and Erica. Theo, Cor, Oliver, Babuna, Chris and Sue. To Pat and Tara, Liz and Larry, Karen and Morgan and Catherine. To Evleyn, Ita and Fiona. To Declan, Brian and Mark. If I have left you out I am sorry and please let me know. To people who I have been inspired by but have never met: Tad James, Richard Bandler, John Grinder, Marilee Goldberg, Milton Erickson and Morihei Ueshiba. To all at Bupa and PPC. To Norman and Pat, Anne, Nellie, Pat and the Moytura crew.

To my clients who encouraged, demanded, insisted, threatened and cajoled me into writing this book.

Thank you.

Preface

It was the year 1997 and I was working as a life coach, using my skills of NLP hypnosis and counselling. My body was not feeling good: Too many times I ate the wrong foods in the wrong amounts. I also ate with lightning speed, barely chewing my food before gulping it down in large quantities. A friend of mine suggested I should clean my body by going on a macrobiotic diet. The diet consisted of organic rice, vegetables, seaweed and the odd bit of fish. I had never before controlled my diet, so it seemed like an interesting challenge.

Part of the diet was chewing. I had to chew my food fifty times a mouthful. After I had finished the diet, I went back onto "normal" food. The chewing habit was by this time ingrained and unconscious. Much to my amazement I was eating about half the amount of food I used to eat, and not only that, but I was doing it automatically. I was also eating more wholesome foods than before and they tasted better than ever.

It was then that I had my epiphany. I knew that when I worked with my clients, trying to get then to stop eating so much and to do more exercise, there was something deeply wrong. Getting them to do things they did not want to do seemed to make things worse. I felt I was forcing the mind, and when the mind is forced to do something in a negative way, it does not co-operate. I now understood that I could help people enjoy their food and eat less of it by training them to chew it thoroughly. That's the answer, I thought. I would no longer help my clients stay on their diets—no longer keep telling them to eat less and exercise more to lose weight. Instead, I would just counsel them to focus on increasing their quality of life. That, after all, is what everybody wants.

I realized that I now had a method that could get people to slim by giving them even more of what they want. Did it work? *Yes*. It worked miracles. Why did it work? Because it was—and is—about instant gratification. My clients were feeling good because of the slimming process itself—which is what this book is all about. I have spent thousands of hours using this process with people who want to lose weight. It has worked for them, and it will work for you. You will also increase your self-esteem and become happier in yourself as you gain a more positive outlook. All you have to do is chew.

I recommend enjoying and chewing food to most of my clients, not only those who want to lose weight. When I am working with clients who need more self-esteem, or who are stressed, I insist on them chewing their food thoroughly. Clients with habit problems or addictions begin to realise that addictions are about being unaware. Chewing their food thoroughly trains them to be in the here and now, where one always has choice.

Imagine if you had never picked up this book and remained caught in the painful self-depreciating cycle of dieting, feeling bad and putting weight back on. Now that you have this book, you can experience yourself more comfortably; you can slim without diets, and with more positive and joyous attitudes towards yourself and your body. Enjoy the book and, while you are reading it, enjoy life as well, by savouring your food and experiencing the pleasure of becoming lighter in body, mind and heart.

Introduction

What is this book all about? It is about eating food the way your body is designed to eat. Why is this method so powerful and successful? Because it is not about the content of eating; it is about the process. In other words, all other slimming methods are about what to eat or what not to eat, which is the content. This book is about *how* to eat, which is the process.

So how do we lose weight? The formula is simple: Eat less food and do more exercise. Basically, this amounts to less energy in, more energy out. What is so complex about that and why, for a lot of us, is it so difficult to do? The answer is our attitude. Instead of being preoccupied with *what* we eat, we need to take a new approach—to food, our bodies and *how* we eat. Of course, what we eat is important, but if we get the process right—how we eat—then it is easy to manage the content—what we eat.

Why this book is for you

This book focuses on three major factors in weight loss: attitude, eating and exercise.

1. Attitude

It seems the world wants to slim, and yet with conventional

methods, we are not doing a good job. Why does it have to be such a struggle? Attitude is a big problem, but not the only one. There is also the problem of how we eat. This book is a complete slimming programme in itself; however, if you are already following a conventional slimming programme, this book will help enhance and accelerate it. The irony is that a successful slimming programme is not based on slimming—it is based on increasing quality of life and happiness.

This book will change your attitude to slimming, eating, food and yourself—you will never look at them the same way again. If you are caught up in the weight-loss cycle of dieting, then putting on weight, then dieting again, here is the answer. If you are in a constant battle with foods you want to eat but cannot, calorie counting, obsessing, punishing then rewarding, loving food and hating it at the same time, bolting your food, eating too much, feeling too hungry and then too full, this book will set you free. The simple methods I will explain are tried and tested; they work, and they will work for you.

2. Eating

How we eat and what we eat *for* are two important processes that have been all but lost in our modern society. We have turned into carnivores, wolfing our food down with the minimum of natural processing. The average amount of chews people give their food is around ten per mouthful. Most people who are overweight chew much less than this. If food is not chewed properly, our bodies become unaware of how much we have ingested.

There are approximately nine thousand taste-buds on the tongue. These little taste-buds act as monitors that count the amount of fats, sugars, salts, proteins and starches that we ingest. When we do not chew, and eat too fast, the taste-buds cannot count how much we ingest, so we eat too much because we are unaware. The body knows how much it needs if we allow it to do its job. Eating too quickly causes physical, emotional and psychological harm.

3. Exercise

The problem with exercising only to slim is that it becomes a form of punishment and loses its purpose. In general, people are either too severe on themselves and fail to exercise because they think they can't do it properly, or they avoid it because it's painful. The focus of exercise needs to be on joy, intelligence and cleaning the body; these are the important by-products of exercise. It is a mistake to exercise solely to slim because it can create negative connotations, which have negative results.

How is your attitude?

Do you jump on the scales more than
once a week?   Yes ___ No ___

Do you count calories?   Yes ___ No ___

Is food on your mind all the time?   Yes ___ No ___

Have you tried several diets and failed?   Yes ___ No ___

Do you feel guilty when you have indulged? Yes ___ No ___

Do you dislike your body or
are you ashamed of it?   Yes ___ No ___

Do you argue with yourself: Will I eat?
Should I eat?   Yes ___ No ___

How do you eat?

Are you a fast eater?	Yes ___ No ___
Do you feel bloated after eating?	Yes ___ No ___

Do you sometimes find you have eaten something
and have been almost unaware of eating it? Yes ___ No ___

Do you eat and drink what is put in front of you—not
the quantity your body chooses? Yes ___ No ___

How is your exercise or body movement?

Do you intend to get exercise but usually
end up not doing it? Yes ___No ___

Do you look on exercise as a chore,
something you have to do? Yes ___No ___

Do you exercise to slim and not
for any other reason? Yes___ No___

Do you feel that exercise is an
unnecessary hardship? Yes ___No ___

If you have answered *yes* to many of these questions, you may be suffering from a negative eating strategy. It is a behaviour you have developed, and behaviour can be changed. This book will show you how.

Why this method? Because it works!

Here is what will happen to you when you take the simple advice offered in this book—without any diets, without any heavy exercise routines or drugs. Too good to be true? No.

1. You will start to feel more relaxed and confident within yourself.

2. You will drop all negative obsessive thinking around food.

3. You will enjoy your food more and eat less.

4. Your body will feel light and you will have more energy.

5. Between one and two weeks, on average, you will start to shed excess weight.

6. You will then feel your clothes loosen.

7. You will continue to shed weight until you have reached your natural slimness; then you will stay there.

8. This is steady, powerful change.

This is what my clients experience; this is what you will experience. It's simple—no starvation diets, no excessive workouts—just follow your body's natural desires.

So why do we slim in the first place?

In some cultures, to have a nice, cuddly, round physique is very desirable. So why are we focused on being slim? It's all to do with the relationship between health and attraction. We are attracted to healthy people of the opposite sex because they will be good for breeding. If they are too skinny and emaciated, they are more likely to be ill. If they are very overweight, they are more likely to be unhealthy. On the overall scale of things, we are better off with the moderately overweight person, as they are more likely to be healthier.

Within the human brain is a part built to recognise the healthy state of people with whom we interact. In general, a man will look for symmetry, and a woman will look for the same. It's health we are after and that's good for our survival. The more symmetrical we are, the more healthy. Whether we are considered to be thin or plump depends on the cultural mores at the time. In a lot of third-world countries, to be plump is attractive; to be thin means poverty or ill health. So if you had a couple of extra kilos and you were in a worldwide beauty contest with a waiflike model, you might be surprised at the outcome. Considering that third-world countries have higher populations, and all the people of the world voted, overall, with a plump body, you would win the vote.

We want to be loved—it is a fundamental part of our survival mechanism, as well as a fundamental part of our happiness. As infants, we know it is important to be noticed to survive. We can make very powerful, irritating sounds when we are ignored. If we are ignored, we die, because we cannot fend for ourselves. As we get older, this infantile need stays with us, even though we are more capable of survival. We get confused between what we think is attraction and love. When we feel attractive, we feel liked; this gives us an instantaneous hit, which is nice, but it is only on a superficial level—a level that is not deep enough to truly nurture us. To a certain extent, wanting to look attractive is normal and healthy, but if we take this desire too far, we develop an unhealthy addiction to trying to look like what we think others find attractive. We have to keep getting superficial approval from others but, even so, we are never satisfied. Like a junky who continues to take a drug, we are never satisfied enough to stop, because the drug cannot reach to the deeper levels of the self.

How are we ever going to be satisfied or feel that we are loved? We can start by remembering that real love is there for everyone, no matter who they are, or what they look like. If only physical attractiveness were the source of love, then a child would not love an overweight, wrinkly grandparent. But in reality, because we love our grandparents, they become attractive. Similarly, what we need to do is to accept ourselves. No matter what we do, or did, we are always doing the best with what we have. That's the human condition. Would you rather be slim and dislike yourself? Or would you rather be a little overweight and like yourself?

Well, I have good news for you. You can like yourself at any weight. But do you want to like yourself and attain your optimum slimness at the same time? Read on . . .

Now answer this question: Just supposing you could only choose between being slim or being happy, which one would you rather be? Think carefully. Put a tick beside the one you choose.

A. I would rather be happy but not slim ____.

B. I would rather be slim but not happy ____.

You know that you can be happy and slim at the same time, but just for this exercise, imagine that you could only be either slim and miserable or plump and happy. If you choose A, then you are on your way to reaching your ideal slimness, and this book is for you. You have a well-balanced ego and will get results fast and easily.

If you answered B, however, you are in troubled waters. Think of what you are choosing. You are saying: "I would rather be slim and miserable than overweight and happy." If you said "Well, if I were slim, I would be happy", and that's why you chose B, then choose again. Imagine you could only choose one, which would you choose? If it is still B, then you must forget all about slimming and work on yourself, for you are most likely experiencing an imbalance in your ego. A good psychologist or psychiatrist may be able to help you. You need to love and accept yourself more.

Not loving yourself suppresses effective motivation and action. It gets you nothing and nowhere. When we do not love or accept ourselves, it is very difficult to change for the better. When we discover self-acceptance, positive change becomes easy. Here is the secret: No matter who you are and what you have done, you have no excuse not to love yourself. This one basic truth is at the heart of sensual—and successful—slimming.

Part I

The Importance of
Attitude

Chapter 1

Attitude: What lies beneath

We become slim by the pursuit of honest-to-goodness joy and happiness, not by the imposition of negativity and punishment.

Our attitude towards food, and towards our bodies and ourselves, is one of the largest factors influencing weight control. Attitude guides the mind and (yes, you guessed it) the mind guides the body. Both mind and body thus operate under the direction of attitude.

Chapter overview

1. Why slimming does not work

A value is a principle that is supported by a number of beliefs. What we value in life determines our drive. If I place a high value on friendship, then I will spend a lot of my time and energy making and being with friends. If I place a low value on wealth, I will spend little time making money. By the same token, slimming is a low value in many people's lives; otherwise, they would have lost weight by now.

2. Towards and away-from attitudes

The focus of our attitudes determines our ability to succeed, not only in weight control but in other areas of our lives as well. We need to make sure our attitudes are directed towards what we want and not merely away from what we do not want.

Accept your body and your condition now. Only then can you change it. Most people who want to slim do not accept themselves or their bodies. They think this non-acceptance will give them motivation to change. But if it did, they would have changed already.

1. Why slimming does not work

Slimming is a low value

Slimming is a low value, because we want to be slim to get something else. We want to be slim to be happy or confident or to feel good. It becomes a problem when we think being slim is the *only way* to feel good, happy, confident and so on. There are many ways to happiness, confidence and feeling good, and they do not require one to be slim.

An effective slimming strategy is not based on slimming. It is based on an increase in quality of life—which is essentially a matter of realising what is actually uplifting, rather than what society, advertising or other people perceive as enjoyable. For example, we might like a light salad and glass of water but if that is all we are going to eat because we feel we are too fat, then we are not going to enjoy it very much. Exercise feels good, but if we exercise because we do not like our bodies the way they are, it is a punishment rather than a pleasure. To be constantly focused on our bodies—negatively obsessed with how we are not looking, comparing ourselves to others, constantly nagging ourselves about food and not enjoying it—is no quality of life.

One of the fundamentals of quality of life is health. Good health means we are comfortable within our bodies and can get a lot of pleasure out of just being fit. It always struck me as interesting that when I worked with clients and elicited their life values, these values were never about being slim. A value, which is usually unconscious, is supported by several beliefs, and it determines our drive. People who are well aligned with their lives give the most time and attention to their top values, and naturally have the motivation to do so. If, instead, we are putting a lot of fret and sweat into being slim, and slimming happens to be of low value, is it any wonder that we don't succeed?

In my work with clients, I have never had *being slim* cited as a high value. Among the top values that people hold are health, happiness, love, relationships, family, career, fun, fulfilment and money. The order of values varies from one person to another, and some people include values that others omit. But I have worked with a lot of clients, and at no time in the values elicitation did I get losing weight named as a top value. Some may have expressed it as a value, but when I compared it to their other values, slimming fell off the end of the board. Try the questions below and you will likely find the same thing.

Suppose you could *only* have either one or the other of the value pairs indicated below. This is important: In order for you to rank your values, answer the following questions as if you could only have one or the other.

Would you rather be slim and unloved or not slim and loved?

Would you rather be slim and miserable or a bit tubby and happy?

Would you rather be slim and have no family or have your family and not be slim?

Would you rather have good friends and not be slim or no friends and be slim?

Would you rather have no career and be slim or not be slim and have a career?

Would you rather be sick and slim or healthy and not slim?

Would you rather have money and not be slim or have no money and be slim?

Would you rather be dull and slim or have plenty of humour and not be slim?

Would you rather have good sex and not be slim or have no sex and be slim? (Yeah, right!)

After answering the questions above, were you surprised to find that you never chose being slim? Are you surprised now that your motivation to become slim is not really that strong after all—not as strong as the value you place on good friends or happiness? All that fret and worry about weight over nothing. Do you now understand why you never reached your goal of being slim? The reason is that there was simply not enough congruent motivation.

Congruent motivation is when the whole mind is focused toward getting something that supports a high value. With congruent motivation you succeed; in fact, you cannot fail. If we link slimming to other values, then it will easily come about. Eating food in the manner for which our bodies are designed produces happiness and health. Exercising our bodies also supports happiness and health, two high values that promote slimming. Eating the correct amount of food and enjoying exercise gives us massive amounts of energy. Doing the opposite takes it away. Almost everything we do is because of happiness and/or peace of mind: for example, we fall in love, buy houses, get promoted, buy nice cars, make friends and keep fit. If we look at the higher intent of all these things, they lead us to happiness and, ultimately, to peace of mind.

Anxiety is caused by *not* focusing on what we truly want. Slimming is not what we truly want, because we are always trying to slim to get something else. Nobody wants to slim *just* to slim—people want to slim to look good, to feel good and to be happy. People slim to be healthy, and when they are healthy, they feel happy. Slimming is always done for another reason besides itself. Therefore, it does not work for its own sake, slimming alone does not make us happy or more loving, slimming makes us slim.

WORTH REPEATING

An effective slimming strategy is not based on weight loss; it is based on increasing quality of life. We slim to get something else.

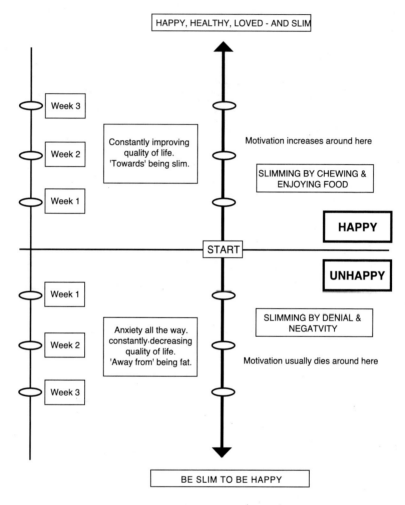

A comparison between the denial methods and the sensual slimming method

The above diagram shows what happens when we put all our effort into slimming and not into health and well-being. Trying to be slim in order to be happy is too indirect for the unconscious mind. We go towards being slim, which is away from our top values of being happy, healthy or loved. Focused only on slimming, we experience anxiety because we are now not focusing on what we truly want. Motivation eventually begins to die, because the mind will not allow us to waste energy on pursuing the low value of being slim. It is not that we lack willpower; it is because we are intelligent that we constantly fail at slimming.

Give yourself a pat on the back if you have failed at slimming through methods of denial and guilt; it means that you are a sane, rational, intelligent human being. The power of focus needs to be directed toward quality of life. We enjoy our food; exercise for feeling good; entertain positive, effective thought habits; and slim in the process. Slimming becomes a side event, achieved while increasing our enjoyment of life. There is a disease whereby a person will reach the slim goal before the happy goal and its called *anorexia nervosa*. Ask the average anorexic "Are you happy?" and if the answer were truthful, it would be: "How could I be happy when I am this obsessive?"

WORTH REPEATING

Give yourself a pat on the back if you have failed at slimming through methods of denial and guilt; it means that you are a sane, rational, intelligent human being.

---

2. Towards and away-from attitudes

The way we look at becoming slim is important. The diagram below shows two different attitudes and how they work. Does the diagram on the right look familiar to you? Simply changing our attitude to weight loss will greatly increase our success.

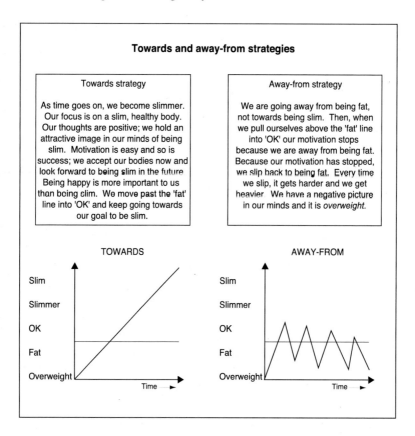

Towards and away-from strategies

Towards strategy

As time goes on, we become slimmer. Our focus is on a slim, healthy body. Our thoughts are positive; we hold an attractive image in our minds of being slim. Motivation is easy and so is success; we accept our bodies now and look forward to being slim in the future. Being happy is more important to us than being slim. We move past the 'fat' line into 'OK' and keep going towards our goal to be slim.

Away-from strategy

We are going away from being fat, not towards being slim. Then, when we pull ourselves above the 'fat' line into 'OK' our motivation stops because we are away from being fat. Because our motivation has stopped, we slip back to being fat. Every time we slip, it gets harder and we get heavier. We have a negative picture in our minds and it is *overweight*.

Towards being slim

The section on the left of the above diagram, entitled "towards", indicates a desirable attitude to slimming. It is positive; people with this attitude keep the rewards in mind and enjoy the process. The graph on the left shows how people can move towards being slim and happy or healthy. As time goes by, they become slimmer. Their primary focus is on health, good feelings and positive feedback. They are being drawn towards their goal. They have a positive mental picture of themselves being slim, and they believe it, but it is not the most important part of their lives. These people accept the way they are now and know they are about to get slimmer.

Away from being fat

The section on the right represents the "away-from" attitude to slimming. While people with this attitude might tell you that they want to be slim, on further questioning you may find they actually do not want to be fat. They are trying to get away from being fat, as opposed to going towards being slim. As time goes on, they often make the same progress as the towards person. Then, after a while, the motivation stops. Why? Because they are no longer fat. They have moved away from being fat and unconsciously have achieved their goal, at least in part. The motivation to keep going thus fails. The problem is that while these people are no longer fat, they are not yet slim either.

Meanwhile, they slide back into their old habits and find themselves fat again. Over time, they get worse and worse. They tend to try and get motivated using negative images of themselves, guilt and negative self-dialogue. They may sometimes have a positive picture in mind, but they don't really believe in it. More likely they carry a stronger picture of the fat body they don't want. They think about it all day long and so programme their bodies to be fat.

The law of reversed effort

The more we want or must have something, the less we get it. When the law of reversed effort comes into play, the more you might want something desperately, the less you get it. This is the classic away-from situation and it is self-perpetuating: The more I want it, the less I get it, so the more I want it, the less I get it, and so on . . . The law of reversed effort is triggered when we are dealing with an away-from mind-set and mistake it for towards. We think we want to go towards being slim when what we really want is to be away from being fat. The more we want to be slim, the fatter we get, because we are thinking about not being fat, instead of being slim. We hate or dislike our bodies for being fat, and the disliking of self freezes the mind, frustrating our effort to get what we want. If we "have to be slim in order to be happy", we usually get the opposite outcome. The unconscious mind is a noble entity—it will not allow us to motivate by negativity in a non safety situation.

Conclusion

Denial and negativity are two powerful processes that work against the practice of slimming. It is a wonder how anyone caught in these processes could succeed. When our values are not aligned with our purpose, it is very difficult to move forward. Slimming is a low value, which is why it is so difficult to succeed at when it becomes the most important issue in our lives. We do not fail at slimming because we are weak willed, but because our minds are rational and balanced. Our mind refuses to give up its power to an insignificant goal. When we align our slimming with high values, such as love, freedom, health and happiness, our minds give power and motivation to these values, and therefore we succeed at slimming. When we have a value that is away from what we do not want, the destination could be anywhere. When we are only trying to get away from being fat, then the motivation stops and we fall back to being overweight again.

Chapter 2

Attitude: How we get what we do not want

Conditional love is not love; it is control. Unconditional love is love and ultimately our true power. Outside conditions of safety negativity kills motivation; positivity enhances it—you choose . . .

Chapter overview

1. Conditional acceptance and denial

(i) When positive motivation does not seem to work, we start using negative motivation

(ii) Negative denial; Positive denial

(iii) Going too far

2. The reverse outcome of a negative attitude

(i) Why negativity does not work

(ii) That which a person hates, or is prejudiced against, has power over them

(iii) Obsession

I. Conditional acceptance and denial

Our attitude towards ourselves is important, there is a noble part in everyone that reacts favourably to positive encouragement. The same part reacts negatively to negative put-downs and conditional acceptance. Unconditional love only please: Self-put-downs, comparisons and conditional acceptance destroy motivation and positivity.

(i) When positive motivation does not work, we start using negative motivation

Negative denial often happens when we treat slimming as a high value, when in fact it is not. We implement ever-stricter diets and force ourselves into an even stronger exercise regime. These tactics, of course, only work on a temporary basis, because motivation is unconsciously reserved for higher values, such as love, health, humour and so on.

When a motivation strategy is not working, then we start to become more negative. We say "I'd better get up or I will be late for work"; then if we snooze, we say it again a little more urgently, until it becomes a shout. We start with a soft "time to get up", and if this does not work, we end up with a "get out of bed, you lazy good-for-nothing". If we have a good quality of life, then a positively toned "time to get up " usually works very nicely. When we have a poor quality of life, there is nothing fantastic to get up to. We usually have to end up shouting negatively at ourselves to get up, which only adds to a poor quality of life.

When motivation becomes negative, then the trouble begins, as we move on to negative denial, conditional rejection and negative communication. From hereon in, to achieve anything is very difficult.

30

CASE HISTORY

A client came to me and she was a little overweight. She explained how she had dieted, lost weight, stopped and put on weight; then she did it all over again. And when she stopped, she put on even more weight than before—the usual sin-guilt-punishment-damnation cycle. She said she was doing just fine; it was tough but she was getting through it. She had been on her latest diet for two weeks and was shedding weight, while fighting hunger in a strict regimen of denial, limiting herself to cabbage soup, salads, lean meats and water.

Her breaking point is a typical example of what this kind of diet does to us. She went into a buffet restaurant to get her black tea and two small triangles of toast, and as she passed the counter, she spotted a big cheesecake. It was one of those cheesecakes, she said, that is made of cream, cream cheese, eggs and sugar, with a crushed sweet biscuit and butter base. She thought to herself, *there is no way I'm having any of that.* When she arrived at the counter to place her order, she said, much to her amazement, "Could I have a cup of black tea, two small triangles of toast and"—here is the reptilian brain stepping in—"a slice of that cheese cake." She nearly clapped her hand over her mouth. It was like some other force took her over and ordered the cheesecake against her will. When she got her tray, she handed money to the cashier and sat down, not even waiting for her change. She devoured the cheesecake and ignored her tea and toast.

She experienced the power of the reptilian brain. In this case there was too much negative denial. We agreed that she would let go of the diet for the time being. The first week she concentrated on chewing her food and tasting each morsel. She said she found it boring at first but then started to really taste and enjoy her food. The next week she started to eat less. I insisted she have three meals a day with the odd snack in between. She then began to go for walks every second day. Within a period of three weeks she was getting lighter. She came to me several weeks later, looking slimmer, and said that she was enjoying life much more. She reported that she had ordered another slice of cheesecake one afternoon. She started eating the cake with relish, really tasting it fully. Much to her delight, she ate some of it and left the rest behind, completely satisfied—a very different feeling than before when she'd eaten the whole thing and felt disgusted with herself.

Attitude is very important. The first thing we need to do is make sure we focus on a positive, towards attitude. We need to accept our bodies as they are now—not wait until they are slim in the future, remember tomorrow never comes. A positive attitude brings positive results; a negative attitude destroys motivation and self-esteem.

(ii) Negative Denial; Positive Denial

Positive denial is a *towards* attitude: I deny myself overindulgence in too many fatty foods because I want to get slim; however, I am a good person. I deny myself extra, unnecessary sleep in the morning, because I want to walk and be fit; but I am a good person whether or not I do so. The difference between positive and negative denial is that negative denial has conditional rejection and guilt—it is aimed at the person by the person. Positive denial is based on encouragement and is aimed at the behaviour, for the person's well-being.

With positive denial, staying in bed is OK—we can rest if we want to and feel good; or we can get up early and do our exercise. We are more likely to get up and exercise because we feel good. If we are overtired, then it is better we rest. The point is: We feel good if we exercise and we feel OK about staying in bed if we need to.

Negative denial goes: "I am a bad, ugly person. I deny myself sleep in the morning because I must get up and punish myself with exercise for being a fat, ugly person. If I feel too tired and don't get up, it's because I am not only an ugly person, but I am also lazy and good for nothing. If I fail, I reject myself and feel guilty; if I get up, I have to punish myself and go for a walk because I am overweight." Here we are again—in a lose-lose situation.

A scold-and-punishment system implies conditional rejection, and conditional rejection reduces motivation. This process also causes weakness in the person, dividing the self into *should* and *should not* rhetoric. People say: "I was good yesterday; I only ate a lettuce leaf and an olive." Or: "I was bad yesterday; I ate cheesecake and a biscuit." People are not good or bad for eating particular types of food. If you follow your body's guidelines, you will eat correctly.

The reward system is unhealthy if it is based on wrong and right. If we reward ourselves for not eating food, it means that eating food is to be avoided. We are good or successful if we do not eat, which can be understood as: We are bad or unsuccessful if we eat. This can produce an anxiety around eating and reinforce the "not there" syndrome.

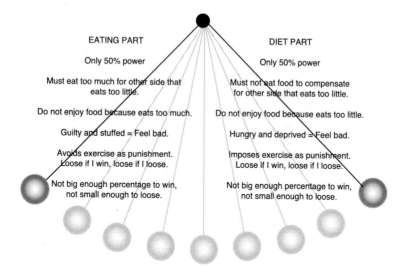

Negative denial and conditional acceptance

The divided, unbalanced self; the losing self. The above diagram is of the divided self, and both sides are always losing. Each side is not big enough to have its way. Here we see the classic negative slimming strategy, dieting and exercising because we are wrong or bad for being fat. By setting up negative denial, we inevitably fail. Whether we eat too much, or do not eat at all, we feel bad. We may "win" temporarily but we always lose in the end.

Positive denial and conditional acceptance

EATING & SATISFACTION IN
HARMONY

100% power

Likes to eat but not too much.
Enjoys food, chews well, likes
the taste and relaxing effect.

Looks forward to eating because
of good feelings and pleasure.

Enjoys exercise as play because
of good feelings.

All parts of the system are
moving in the same direction.

Always win-win.

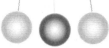

Positive denial and unconditional acceptance

The united, balanced self—the winning self. Here we have the united self. There is no guilt around eating food, so we are free to eat and enjoy it. We also like exercise because exercise is enjoyable—it gives us good feelings. We become slim by the pursuit of joy and happiness, not by the imposition of negativity and punishment. We accept ourselves unconditionally and see the process of enjoying food: eating enough but not too much, and exercising because it feels good.

(iii) Going too far

With severe negative denial we awaken the survival mechanism of the brain. This is our most powerful drive—it will override rational control and make us eat. If we starve ourselves to become slim, the survival mechanism prompts us to eat food to restore the balance—hence, the bingeing process. When the survival mechanism drives us to do something against our will, it is called *temporary insanity* in legal terms. I have worked with borderline anorexics who have reported blackouts of consciousness, only to awaken fisting food into their mouths. That is the work of a healthy survival mechanism. Negative denial causes dangerous internal conflict. We force ourselves onto a starvation diet for a while, but inevitably (if we are emotionally healthy) we break out and eat. Sound familiar?

2. The reverse outcome of negative attitude

The mind is a highly complex system but it works on simple principles—when we use negative language and imagery, it produces negative results. We often make the mistake of trying to motivate ourselves with too much negativity. Effective thinking produces effective results. Get rid of negative language, guilt and negative imaging. They make us fat.

The inner mind processes positives first and negatives after wards. If we make a picture of ourselves as overweight and we say "not that", the mind will just bring us towards the picture of being overweight. Read this:

"Don't think of a red door."

What did you think of as you read that? That's right: a red door. If we say "I don't want to be fat", we are saying to ourselves "Be fat". Our unconscious mind processes the positive first and negatives second, but by then it is too late. An away-from pattern involves wanting something while thinking about what we do *not* want. In other words, we say "I want to be slim", but we are making a picture of getting away from a FAT BODY. So FAT BODY is programmed into the unconscious mind and we go towards being fat. The towards strategy is "I want to be slim because it's nice to BE SLIM", and we make a picture of ourselves being slim. The message to the unconscious is highlighted in capitals—the same as "Don't think of A RED DOOR."

Whatever we make an image of, or think about, our minds will go and get it for us—that's their job. The part of the mind that operates at this level does not consider what is good or bad for us—it just goes towards what we think about. The mind is a guided system and the system is guided by whatever we present to the mind in words or images. If we are thinking about food all day, what do we command our minds to do? Yes, get food. Remember that the inner mind processes positives first. If I am thinking of not eating food, I'm still programming in: *Eat food.* (Don't think of a red door . . . Oh, too late.) Remember the towards and away-from principles.

The reason why the old conventional slimming processes do not work is because they break some fundamental rules. Most slimming and weight-loss programmes used to hinge on methods of denial, conditional acceptance, being good or bad, unnatural food-stuffs and calorie counting. What does this do? That's right: It focuses us on food all day. What does the mind do then? Yes, yes—it directs us towards eating.

If we jump on the scales every day and worry about what we are, or are not, going to eat—if we calorie count, fight with food, fight with ourselves to eat less, and dislike our bodies because they are fat—we are programming the body to eat and be fat. That's why negativity actually works in the opposite direction. So stop now.

(i) Why negativity does not work

What if a child came up to us and asked, "What do you think

of my drawing of a cat?"—and we saw scrawled on a piece of paper something remotely resembling a cat? Imagine the impact on the child if we said, "That is terrible; it hardly resembles a cat; you need several years training before you can even draw. You are useless, no good, and you look awful."

How do you think that child would feel now? Do you think the child would be motivated to draw after that? I don't think so. Yet we do the same thing when we are down on ourselves all day long and then wonder why we do not do anything about our weight. Stop the negative self-dialogue of self-dissatisfaction. No matter how much we scold ourselves, argue, cajole and compare, this only decreases, and never increases, motivation. We must stop. We might think: *But if we stop, then we won't do anything about losing weight.* In fact, however, if we like ourselves, we keep ourselves healthy and slim. If there are things we would like to change, it is much more efficient to change in a direction that we can enjoy as we change. So if a child shows us a picture of a cat, no matter how simple, we say, "Oh, that's beautiful—what a lovely picture. You are really talented; you are a wonderful person; look at how well you draw; you are getting better and better the more you practise."

How do you think the child will feel now—motivated? Yes, and encouraged to do better next time. The child knows full well that its picture and the real thing are far apart, but to a child that does not matter; they thrive on encouragement just like adults. A four- or five-year-old child only has so much dexterity in their hands. They are doing the best they can—and so are you.

The Ineffective Parent		The Effective Parent
"That is a hopeless drawing of a cat; it's stupid, innacurate, no good. You are useless, good for nothing and you cant't draw; you never do anything right; you're bad."		"That's a wonderful drawing; you will make a great artist with practice. You are a good person capable of wonderful things; you are magnificent."

Negativity kills motivation and destroys creativity.

If we say to ourselves "Go on a diet, you fat idiot; you're useless; look at you—can't even wear clothes anymore; you're lazy and good for nothing . . .", do we now feel good? And would anyone ever feel successful after such a put-down? Do we feel like doing something to reduce weight now? I don't think so. Self-dialogue with sentences like *I must, I should, I should not, I have to, I need to, I must not* and *I must* stress the mind. These particular messages can cause panic within the system and, to a certain degree, stress the individual. If a person is under too much stress, they are even less motivated than normal.

(ii) That which a person hates, or is prejudiced against, has power over them

When we hate, dislike, or are prejudiced against something, it has power over us. If I am afraid of spiders, then all someone has to do is produce one to get control over me:

"If you don't give me what I want, I will bring out the spider."

"Oh no, please, anything but the spider."

39

It is the same thing with people. When we dislike or hate another person, that person now has control over us. The one I dislike does not have to do anything to me: Just thinking about the person causes my blood chemistry to change. I have given my power away—that's what dislike or hate does.

It is the same thing with ourselves. If we do not like part of ourselves (the part that eats too much or the body that results), we have now increased the power of that part by disliking it (so we eat even more and the body puts on more weight). This happens because rejecting or judging something, or somebody, cuts off communication, and without communication, there is no reconciliation. The situation becomes stuck, and we are left with anxiety. Even when there is conflict, if we stay open and accepting we can resolve the issues between us and people or things—which then become ordinary and no longer have any negative effect. One example is when we make up and forgive.

In no situation is it ever a good idea to give our power away and waste our resources disliking, hating or judging negatively. So many of my clients come in with weight problems because they dislike the part of them that eats, and they dislike their bodies. Both of these parts are completely innocent. If they dislike parts of themselves, those parts become fixed and very difficult to change. The eating part eats more, and the "don't want to exercise" part wins out every time.

All the sages tell us that love is the true power, not specifically as a way of getting into heaven or nirvana or of becoming enlightened (although it probably helps), but as a very effective way of moving through the world. If you do not hate things, people, behaviours or your own personality, then you are a person at peace with yourself. Acceptance is the forerunner of intelligent change.

The secret to slimming is to move as a united self, towards quality of life that will cause the slimming to happen as a beneficial side effect. We are always trying to move in a main direction, and that is towards more quality of life. Peace of mind and happiness are always more important than losing a few pounds.

CASE HISTORY

One of my clients started the programme. After about two weeks, he was chewing his food at least forty times a mouthful. He was eating far less food and enjoying it much more. He had increased his exercise and was really liking it. He was enjoying food for its own sake and enjoying exercise for its own sake, a perfect combination. He shed a little weight but then stopped with about two stone to go and did not lose any more. This was a great puzzle to me as he was then defying the laws of physics. Less energy into his body, and more energy out, means his body has to become lighter.

> I sat opposite him in my office and then, intuitively, I asked him, "How do you feel about your body?" He looked distracted all of a sudden and then said, "I hate my body; it's fat and ugly looking." That was it. I worked with the client throughout that whole session to help him with accepting his body. After that, the client shed all excess weight. To dislike your body is to dislike yourself—your body is your mind; your mind is your body. Accept your body. It is reacting intelligently to your behaviour; there is nothing wrong with your body.
>
> Fat is a quick, temporary coating stored on the outside; it is excess energy. Our skeletal structure has not changed; we are always slim inside.

(iii) Obsession

Obsession begins when a person's life now revolves around denial of, and conflict with, food, with the focus away from being fat. When we are in this type of thinking, we have become obsessive.

Food, dieting and not being fat take up over 40 percent of our thoughts. Each thought is programming our bodies to become fat. While we are thinking about being fat, we are trying to be slim; the mind is torn in two; obsession increases and so does weight.

Here are some indicators that you may be getting dangerously close to obsession:

> ➢ Thinking about what you can and cannot eat all day long.
> ➢ Feeling anxious when you are invited to a social event where there is food.
> ➢ Jumping on the scales more than once a week.

- Having low-fat spreads, drinks and sweeteners, even though you would enjoy real ones.
- Constantly comparing your body to others.
- Constantly talking about food, eating or not eating.
- Beating yourself up negatively about how much you do and do not eat.
- Beating yourself up negatively about your body.
- Beating yourself up regularly about what a bad person you are if you have eaten too much.
- Using words like *bad* or *good* when describing eating or not eating.
- Feeling guilty if you eat.
- Feeling miserable if you do not eat.

This kind of obsessive thinking leads to an overweight body or a severely underweight body. The irony is that the thought processes of someone who is struggling with obesity and one who is struggling with anorexia nervosa are the same. They become self-obsessed. Imagine all the wonderful things to think about and do in this magnificent world, while overweight and underweight people are stuck, suffering, looking down at their own bodies, feeling bad, while the world and its wonders pass them by.

WORTH REPEATING

Imagine all the wonderful things to think about and do in this magnificent world, while overweight and underweight people are stuck, suffering, looking down at their own bodies, feeling bad, while the world and its wonders pass them by.

What if I choose to keep my negative attitude to slimming?

1. I may not achieve a better quality of life.
2. I will be miserable with myself.
3. I will have low self-esteem and confidence.
4. I will have an unhealthy body.
5. I will struggle for the rest of my life.

What if I choose a positive attitude towards slimming?

1. I will achieve a better quality of life.
2. I will be a happier person.
3. My self-esteem and confidence will be higher.
4. I will have a healthy body.
5. I will be free for the rest of my life.

Conclusion

Attitude is important. When we have away-from attitudes—negative denial, conditional rejection and negative language and imagery—there is no slimming method in heaven or on earth that is going to work effectively. We can go on all the diets we like—go to all the personal coaches, trainers, dieticians and health farms—they will not work. It all starts with the mind. The idea is to turn your ultimate focus towards increasing your quality of life. Why waste all that energy and thought on misery and worry about eating and fat? You know you are much more than that. The process of slimming with a positive, *towards* attitude causes you to increase your quality of life, making you a stronger, more emotionally balanced person. The fundamental element of this process is unconditional love, the most powerful force in the universe; and because of this, you will succeed.

Part II

Mind, Body and Eating

Chapter 3

Your Mind and the Process of Eating

He who distinguishes the true savour of his food can never be a
glutton; he who does not cannot be otherwise.
—Henry David Thoreau

*Unless we get the process (how to eat) right, there is little chance
of getting the content (how much and what to eat) right.*

The reason why the sensual slimming method is so powerful is
that it is about the process (how we eat) and not the content (what we
eat). Conventional slimming programmes are all caught up with what
to eat—the content—which is why they are only partially successful.
Focusing on the content and not the process is putting the cart before
the horse. Unless we get the process (how to eat) right, there is little
chance of getting the content (how much and what to eat) right. How
do we put on weight? Simple—by being unaware of our feelings and
eating like carnivores. If, on the other hand, we get in touch with our
bodies, they will let us know how much we need. It is important to be
kind and good to ourselves, and this does not include stuffing food
into our bodies. Eating too fast causes eating too much. Most people
in our society eat too fast and too much—and they do so with too
little sensual awareness.

Chapter overview

1. Sensitivity

If we are sensitive to what our bodies' sophisticated feedback systems are telling us, then we no longer have a problem. Our mouths have a sophisticated detection system to monitor the amount of salts, sugars and fats that enter our system. These detection systems are our taste-buds. There are around nine thousand of them, and for good reason.

2. The "not there, don't care" syndrome

How do we overeat? By being out to lunch when we are out to lunch. It is important to be in the now when we eat. Many people who eat too much are generally not there while they eat; it is as though food is just something to dump into the body with a "get rid of it" attitude. The "not there" syndrome is when we eat but our minds are on something completely different.

3. Eat the way our bodies are designed to eat

If we eat the way our bodies are designed to eat, we will take in just enough to be healthy and slim. We are omnivores, and omnivores are supposed to eat in a way that supports the health of their bodies. There is no point in eating like a herbivore or carnivore, because that is not a healthy way to eat for our bodies.

1. Sensitivity

If we are sensitive to what our bodies' sophisticated feedback systems are telling us, then we no longer have a problem. Our mouths have a sophisticated detection system to monitor the amount of salts, sugars and fats that enter our system. These detection systems are our taste-buds. By chewing our food well, we release all the fats, salts, sugars, proteins and starches across our tongue. Our taste-buds count the amount of food-stuff entering the body and signal to the brain when we have ingested enough. It reacts by turning down the satisfaction we are getting from the food-stuff.

Ninety-nine percent of clients coming to me for weight loss eat too fast. This is not surprising: While my clients are healthy, intelligent, strong-willed people, they have not succeeded at weight loss, and it therefore stands to reason that they are doing something that is not working for them. The secret, plain and simple, is: They have forgotten how to eat.

There are nine thousand or so taste-buds in our mouths. These marvellous little pleasure-seekers have the job of monitoring the amounts of salts, fats, sugars, proteins and starches coming into the body. We don't have to count calories or watch what we eat: Taste-buds do that for us. Leave it up to the experts—it is their job and they do it remarkably well, if we give them a chance. To enable them to do their job, we need to chew our food well to release the fats, salts and sugars. When we eat our food too fast without chewing completely, our taste-buds cannot monitor the amount of food we take in. The food does not stay in the mouth long enough for the taste-buds to do their job. We then ingest too much, or we try to calculate with our eyes or a diet book or a calorie counter, instead of relying on our highly advanced, efficient, effective, taste-buds.

What is healthy and what is not? If we do not know, then this is usually caused by lack of sensitivity. Not knowing how much to eat is like saying "I don't know when I'm too cold" or "I don't know when I'm too hot." It is as if we went out in the snow wearing shorts and a t-shirt for a few hours, turned blue and didn't know it, because we couldn't feel it. On the other hand, imagine going outside in summer, wearing a winter coat when the temperature is 30 Celsius; we'd be sweating like mad and still not even know we were hot. If we were to do these things, there is a good chance we would become ill, even in minor temperature changes. Yet we routinely take a similar risk when we eat too much food.

How do we lose our capacity to recognise what food does, and does not, do? How do we become unaware of our capacity to feel satisfied and only know when we have eaten too much? We can ignore sensitivity by overriding the stimulus many times, until we become unaware of it.

When it gets a little cool, we put on something warm or turn on the heat. When we get too hot, we shed clothing or turn on the air conditioner. We have the same sensitivity when it comes to food, so why do we ignore it and eat too much? Because we eat too fast.

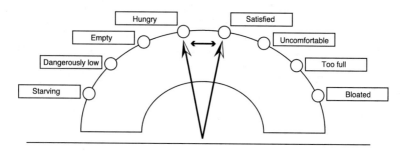

Balanced eating

Normal healthy eater. Above is a diagram of the normal eater. People in this group get hungry and then they eat and feel satisfied. They don't see the point in eating any more than is necessary because, when they do, they feel uncomfortable.

Imagine this is a gage in the brain with a needle that continues moving all day from satisfied to hungry. The above diagram depicts a normal eating strategy. The person feels hungry, eats what is needed and then is satisfied. Many hours later, the needle moves down to hungry and the person again eats until the needle reaches satisfied and stops—and on and on goes this balanced eating cycle.

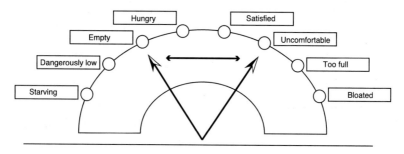

The yo-yo diet. Unbalanced eating leads to overweight.

The above diagram is one of a negative eating strategy. The constant moving from bloated or too full to too hungry wears out the body's natural sensitivity and ability to recognise how much we need to eat for satisfaction. People in this group deny themselves food, until they get very, very hungry; then they eat too much and become too full.

The "skip breakfast" scenario. We need to eat regularly, not have large time-spans between meals, as these only pull the indicator towards the too-hungry mark. Then, when we go to eat, the indicator springs powerfully towards "too full". In the rush to feed ourselves, we miss the mark. "Too hungry" is therefore a bad place to be because it easily leads to "too full". When we skip breakfast, hunger catches up with us later on, usually towards evening time: We are by then too hungry and thus eat until we are too full—which often causes us to skip breakfast—and so on . . .

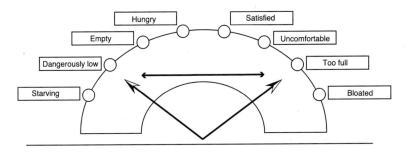

Dangerous dieting leads to psychological and physiological problems.

The binger or bulimic—the wider the swings, the worse the problem: The person above is very out of control. There is almost no enjoyment in eating food; the person is very insensitive to the body's needs. Here is starvation, and then overeating, on a pathological level.

What is natural sensitivity?

Lack of sensitivity: Too little food. Not being sensitive to our bodies' needs so that we eat too little. Starving ourselves to be thin. These reactions are usually in response to previously eating too much food.

We Ignore. Our body's cry for food and pleasure from eating.

We Deny. That we need a proper amount of food to survive healthily.

We Punish. We feel we are in the wrong for our bodies being the way they are.

Lack of sensitivity: Too much food. In this scenario we eat too much—far beyond what our bodies need. We eat until we feel uncomfortably full, and we eat without really tasting our food. This scenario is usually caused by a reaction to too little food.

We Ignore. Our body's cry for us to stop putting too much into our system.

We Deny. That we are taking in too much and that this is causing physical discomfort.

We Punish. We chide ourselves with negative self-talk about our bodies putting on weight.

Sensitivity: Enough food. We eat what feels right. As we eat slowly and purposefully our sensitivity guides us. If we eat foods that are dense (fat saturated), we eat less, and if we eat foods that are light (salads), we eat more.

We Enjoy. We savour our food and get good feelings out of eating.

We Quantify. We automatically eat the right amount of food to run the body healthily.

We Love. Eating the right amount is caring for the self; it increases our self-respect.

2. The "not there, don't care" syndrome

How do we overeat? By being out to lunch when we are out to lunch. It is important to be in the now when we eat. Many people who eat too much are generally not there while they eat; they are looking at their food to get it into the body as if eating demanded a "get rid of it" attitude. The "not there" syndrome is when we eat but our minds are on something completely different. If we are eating and thinking of work, then we are "not there" while eating. If we are eating and tasting, chewing, enjoying and feeling the food, then we are fully present—we are in the "here and now". Sometimes we choose to be "not there" while we eat because we think that eating is making us fat. We don't like to face the problem, so we distract ourselves by being or thinking about anything other than what we are doing. When we are eating, we "get it over with". The "get it over with" problem occurs when we look at the plate of food and think: OK, I have to get all that inside me now, and get it over with. So we stuff in the food, unaware of the tastes, textures, enjoyment and, of course, the amount. We also do it in double-quick time, to get away from the problem. But food is never the problem; the problem is our attitude towards it. Food is a friend; when you are in its company, enjoy it.

If we are not there, then we cannot relax or enjoy our food. The body cannot monitor what it needs, so we eat too much—sometimes the wrong food. If you eat with the attitude of "get it over with", you will stress the body and the mind. The "not there" syndrome is partially responsible for insensitivity: How can we be sensitive to what we are eating if we are not there? And how can we know when we are eating too much?

(i)   We eat food to get rid of it; instead of letting our mouths and stomachs decide, we let our eyes decide how much to eat.

(ii) We eat fast, not chewing our food thoroughly.

(iii) Our mind is everywhere but in the here and now.

(iv) We are not enjoying our food, just throwing it into our bodies.

(v)   We eat supersaturated fatty or sugary foods; because we eat so fast, they are the only foods we can taste.

It is important to be in "the now" when we eat. Give yourself a present of the present. Being present makes it easier to chew our food well, take our time and only ingest what we need. Imagine if you were making love while thinking about work: I think your partner would begin to feel alone. When we are doing one thing while thinking of another, we do not do well.

When we eat too fast, or too much, it is a sure signal that we are unaware of what we are doing and unaware of how we feel. Lots of my clients have reported how they have never been aware of the uncomfortable feelings of eating too much and too fast. They report that after they have developed the habit of chewing food thoroughly, they would not go back to the old way, simply because it feels physically and emotionally uncomfortable. They have become aware of what their body needs.

The taste-buds, our marvellous little pleasure monitors that keep track of the amount of food we eat, need to be able to do their job. They can do their job well if we chew our food thoroughly and are aware of what we are doing. If we put a tablespoon of pure sugar into our mouths and begin to chew it, the sweetness becomes too much as the taste-buds register overwhelming amounts of sugar, and we spit the sugar out. Our bodies have to do this because too much sugar can damage or even kill us, as can too much salt or fat. However, most of us with weight problems eat so fast, all the while "not there", that our taste-buds do not have time to monitor the amount and type of food that we are eating. It is easy to be aware of too much if the food is in concentrated form, like a large spoonful of sugar, fat or salt. It is not that easy if the sugar or fat is diluted among other ingredients. Most people would eat a confectionery bar, but if we placed the ingredients separately on the table in front of them, most would not. Imagine separate piles of cocoa, sugar, fat, salt and preservatives. When combined, they taste good but we often eat so fast we do not allow our taste-buds to count the amounts of sugars and fats; we therefore eat the whole thing when all we needed was a couple of bites.

Imagine you wanted to count out a hundred sheep from a large herd, and your dog rounded them up and then chased them through a wide gap in the fence. The sheep are coming so fast that they rush through the gap in a large chaotic mass. They would be very difficult to count in this way, all rushing through, and we would probably miss a few. At the end of the day, we might well have many more sheep than a hundred.

Similarly, when we eat food too fast, our taste-buds do not have enough time to monitor the amount coming into our bodies, and we may end up with more food than we had intended.

To count sheep we need to take time; it is better that we make a small gap in the fence so that they come through one at a time and that way we can easily count them. It is better, too, that we do not rush or panic them—this makes counting them much less stressful. Now we can accurately know how many sheep we let through the gap.

It is also better for us to eat slowly and meditatively, so that our taste-buds can monitor the amount of foods going into the body and we do not get stressed. In this way, we taste the food and can feel more satisfied with less. Going out to enjoy a nice meal in a favourite restaurant is pointless if we bolt our food: There is no enjoyment in rushing and stressing.

We need to eat the way the body is designed to eat. In this way, we allow our bodies' sophisticated monitoring systems for ingestion to work. Our bodies know how much we need, but they cannot work if we eat too fast. Chew food: Human beings should only swallow fine soup—food has to pass through a membrane to get into the body. Chew food thoroughly: Otherwise we wear out the body.

3. Eat the way our bodies are designed to eat

If we eat the way our bodies are designed to eat, we will eat just enough to be healthy and slim.

We are omnivores, and omnivores are supposed to eat in a way that supports the health of their bodies. There is no point in eating like a herbivore or carnivore, because that is not a healthy way to eat for our bodies. There is no point in carnivores eating like herbivores or omnivores because they are designed to be radically different.

Carnivore	Omnivore	Herbivore
Dog Cat Lion	YOU	Cow Horse Rabbit Deer
(Meat Eater)	(Eats meat & plants)	(Eats plants)
One heavy meal every day or every few days.	Eats food every few hours.	Eats food all day long.
Does not have cheeks or lateral jaw movement Sharp teeth to slice food.	Has cheeks and lateral jaw movement. Molars to grind food down.	Has cheeks and lateral jaw movement. Large molars to grind down food.
Short digestive system.	Medium-length digestive system.	Long digestive system.

A good reason to chew food is that you are an omnivore, halfway between a carnivore and a herbivore. A carnivore is an animal that primarily eats meat. A herbivore is an animal that eats plants. An omnivore is an animal that eats both meat and plants. We are a successful species because we exploit two food sources: plants and animals. Our digestive system has evolved to cope with a variety of foods. We can eat meat and plants and thus have a broad menu. A cat has to eat meat; if its environment has no meat to eat, it dies. A human will in this case simply start eating plants and survive. If a horse cannot get plants or grass in its environment, it dies. A human will start to eat meat (the horse). The carnivore part of the system allows us to eat high-energy food like meat, though we would find it difficult to digest bone or hide—we are not completely adapted to eating meat like a wolf is, for example.

We can eat vegetables and fruit, grains and beets, but we cannot digest leaves, grass or tree bark like a herbivore. We don't have to eat all day like a herbivore, and we cannot survive easily on eating once every three or four days like a large carnivore. We need to eat every day several times, but not continuously. We need to eat soft food, not as hard as leaves and grass or hide and bone. We need to chew this food very, very finely to be able to prepare it for our unique digestive system. A human being needs to swallow food chewed to the consistency of fine soup. Our bodies are designed to swallow liquid food, because this is correct for our digestive system, our health and our psychological well-being.

WORTH REPEATING

A human being needs to swallow food chewed to the consistency of fine soup. Our bodies are designed to swallow liquid food.

A herbivore has a longer digestive system because of the coarseness of its food; a carnivore has a shorter system. Our small intestine is on average twenty-five feet long while, in comparison, a horse's small intestine is eighty-nine feet. A cow has four stomachs to digest grass, which is a coarse, low-quality food; cows also regurgitate the grass, re-chew it and swallow it again. We do not have a long digestive system or four stomachs, and we do not re-chew our food. We have only one chance to break down the food for our systems, so we need to chew and chew well.

Most people eat like carnivores and wonder why they have problems with ulcers, irritable bowl, acid stomachs, wind, weight and so forth. They do not eat according to their system. Our bodies are designed to guide us to eat certain foods at certain times in certain quantities. Let our bodies guide us. We need to remember that our system takes time to react, and it can be slower than our taste-buds. If we wait until our stomachs feel we have had enough, the chances are we have had too much. When we chew food thoroughly, our taste-buds signal directly to the brain; the brain then signals to us when we have had enough by turning down the taste of the food. When the taste is no longer enjoyable, stop eating. In other words, when the food suddenly seems like a bit of a chore to continue eating, stop. This is more efficient and accurate than waiting for our stomachs to feel satisfied.

WORTH REPEATING

When we chew food thoroughly, our taste-buds signal directly to the brain; the brain then signals to us when we have had enough by turning down the taste of the food. When the taste is no longer enjoyable, stop eating.

Eat the way your body and mind are designed to eat.

Chew, chew, chew.

1. Chew your food. As human beings, we should only swallow
    fine soup. We need to chew each mouthful at least forty
    times before swallowing; if it is a tough food, we need to
    chew it up to fifty times or more. Yes, that is why we have
    rows of powerful molars and a bite than has strength up to
    125 pounds per square inch.

Relax.

2. When you place food in your mouth, relax, chew, and rest
    your arms; every so often, put your fork or spoon or sandwich
    down. It is not good if the next morsel of food is hovering
    outside our mouths like a SWAT team ready to burst in.

Be there.

3. Put reasonably sized portions of food in your mouth, the size
    of half the length of your thumb. Be in the now, be fully
    present and conscious—this allows your mind to calm and
    your body to de-stress. Take at least twenty minutes to eat a
    meal.

Taste.

4. Taste the food; be here now. Make a mental note of the tastes
    and textures of the food. Take as much satisfaction out of the
    food as you can—that's what it is there for. Eventually, the
    taste will change, and when this happens, stop eating; it is
    your brain telling you that you have had enough.

It takes twenty minutes after we start eating for our stomachs to
register how much food the body is taking in. If we are in the habit
of eating all our meals in less than this time, we are in danger of
overeating. There is a more sensitive and reactive monitor of food,

and that is the action of our taste-buds. Chew food forty times per mouthful; allow your taste-buds to count, not your eyes or the feeling in your stomach. Our brain can register satisfaction a lot sooner than the stomach if we allow it to taste the food. Let your body decide what it does, or does not, need.

Get into the joy and ceremony of nurturing. Relax and let the sensitivity of your body guide you. In this way, you will start to eat just enough and then you will naturally slim. We need a lot of food if we are physically active, just like an athlete does. However, if we are less active, we need less food.

When we stuff food, and too much of it, into ourselves too quickly, we decrease our sense of self-esteem—we actually fall out with ourselves.

EATING TOO FAST IS LIKE . . .

Imagine you have a good friend whom you love very much. Imagine you go and get a really expensive manicure with French polish on your fingernails. Now the beautician tells you that you cannot touch anything for twelve hours. A while later you are hungry, but you cannot eat because you cannot use your hands. So you call your friend. Your friend says, "Oh, come in, you poor thing, I will cook for you and feed you."

You sit down and wait with positive expectancy for the food to arrive. Finally, your friend puts down a big plate of food in front of you and says "ready?" And with glee, you say "yes".

Then your friend proceeds to ram the food into your mouth in huge lumps; before you have time to swallow, she is ramming the next morsel in. You cannot even say "stop", because she is shoving it in so quickly. Then she gets the dessert in her fist and rams it into your mouth as well. She then grabs you, pulls you to your feet and shoves you out the door, saying "Come back when you want your next meal."

Do you think you would come back?

What would you think of your friend and how would you feel about her now?

In order to treat someone like this, how would you need to feel about that person?

Your answers to the above questions are how you think and feel about yourself inside when you eat too fast. Yet this is what we do to ourselves when we overeat. Is it any wonder our self-esteem takes a blow when we treat ourselves like this? You are much better than that. Eat lovingly, and you and your body will lighten. Eating fast is abusive to the body and mind. Eating too fast erodes self-esteem and self-respect. Eating slowly and enjoying food increases self-respect; chewing our food thoroughly increases self-esteem and unconditional love.

Conclusion

The process of eating is all-important. We know what is healthy food and what is not. Our problem is not ignorance about which foods to eat; our problem is not knowing how to eat food. Our digestive systems, our social makeup and our brain functioning are designed to chew food thoroughly and enjoy taste. We are not carnivores, we are not herbivores—we are omnivores. Our physical equipment is for chewing, enjoying and relaxing with food. Our bodies are designed with the sensors to tell us when we are eating too much. Our attention needs to be inside our bodies when we eat—aware of taste, feelings and pleasure—not outside and away, resisting our senses, scolding ourselves and bolting our food.

Chapter 4

Your Body and the Process of Eating

The body and mind are a system;
everything that we do affects all of that system.

Chapter overview

1. What happens in the digestive system when we eat effectively

2. What happens to the digestive system when we eat too fast

This chapter is about the process of eating, or *how* we eat; it is about what happens in our mouths, stomachs and brains as we eat. If we get the process right, the content will adjust itself, automatically, to our benefit.

I. What happens in the digestive system when we eat effectively

The average person eats up to fifty tonnes of food in a lifetime. We have a marvellous system to deal with the absorption and processing of food. This system is called our digestive system. Below is a simple description of what happens in each phase to each related part of the body.

The mouth

The person chews food thoroughly; human beings should only swallow fine soup. While chewing thoroughly, the person tastes the food and enjoys its textures and sensations. The food is mixed with mucus and saliva and becomes finely ground and slushy. The actual volume of the food increases because more saliva is mixed with the food when processed in this way. From the table to the hand to the mouth—this is the conscious part of eating. The rest is unconscious; the body's automated digestive system looks after it. The approximately nine thousand taste-buds in the mouth start counting the calories as the food is broken down for digestion. If the food is too saturated with fats or sugars, the mouth will alert us and we will eat less because the chewing process allows the taste-buds to monitor the amounts of fats and sugars. The mouth is very important; the more that is done there, the better it is for the rest of our digestive systems.

The Stomach

The stomach secretes acids onto the chewed foods and breaks down the food even more. The food stays an average of three to four hours in the stomach. It leaves the stomach due to a change in the acidity, which causes the sphincter muscle to open; then it enters the small intestine. The pylorus, the exit part of the stomach, only allows food with a diameter of one to two millimetres to pass through it. If the food is too big, it gets thrown back and digested more. Un-masticated food is hard on the stomach; it ages the body. If the food is still too lumpy, the pylorus widens and food has to be shunted out of the stomach by a process known as the "migrating motor complex", which is a clearing mechanism. When we chew our food thoroughly, the stomach does not have to work hard and the food is easily processed. The food is eaten at a much slower rate so that when the twenty-minutes time-span is up, the stomach signals to the brain how much it needs to be satisfied. Bloating or stuffing is avoided. The stomach is happy to retain the food for longer as no clogging takes place. Our stomachs do not suffer from too much acid and we can relax and feel comfortable. Food may stay a little longer in the stomach as a result of chewing well, and we are therefore satisfied for longer.

The small intestine

This is a long tube of twenty-five feet, with a surface area equivalent to four tennis courts. The food is absorbed across a membrane, which takes quite a lot of energy. Here the food is mixed with other digestive body juices and parts of it are absorbed into the body. The food takes up to three hours to move through the small intestine.

When we chew our food well, the bolus, or packet of food, is of a much more slushy, slippery consistency. It moves though the intestine effortlessly; there are large parts of the intestine that are free of food. The intestine absorbs the nutrients easily because they are properly processed, cutting down on fatigue and keeping the system young and healthy.

The large intestine

The large intestine reabsorbs water from the digested food, up to a gallon a day. Food can remain here from eighteen hours to two days. Chewing our food thoroughly prevents irritable bowel. The food is at its proper consistency and therefore does not clog or crimp the large intestine. Many of my clients reported irritable bowel simply clearing up altogether when they started chewing their food.

The brain

The brain experiences the relaxed, intimate process of sensual eating and secretes feel-good chemicals, called endorphins, into the system. The person is self-nurturing in a relaxed, loving way and self-esteem is strengthened. The system starts to relax and de-stress; the mind calms and the person becomes balanced. The person then becomes satisfied and does not need to eat any more for hours. The person enjoys food more and eats less.

This natural eating habit is encoded in our DNA. Our digestive systems are designed to process finely masticated food. Eating is supposed to be a sacred activity—meditative—we are "with" ourselves. We are nurturing ourselves not only physically but mentally and emotionally as well.

2. What happens to the digestive system when we eat too fast

Lets look at the digestive process again, but this time we will consider what happens to the system when we eat too fast. It seems to be a universal problem—everywhere around us, people eat too fast. We see people in pubs and restaurants and at dinners, all eating too fast—wolfing the food down like starving animals. Our bodies are not designed to eat lumpy food; we are not designed physically, mentally and emotionally to eat food fast.

It all starts at the beginning, the mouth or, you could say, even before that—with the attitude. Nowadays, people do not seem to take time to eat food; they have lost the art and ceremony of nurturing. Our lifestyles have become fast, convenient and unhealthy. Most people eat too fast. They ram the food into their mouths, give it a couple of chews, just enough so that it fits down the throat, and then they swallow. This bolting of food gives rise to a whole host of problems, such as ulcers, irritable bowel, heartburn, abdominal and intestinal discomfort. In many cases, this is the symptom of a much greater affliction: not knowing how to care for the self. Not knowing how to care for the self damages the self-esteem of the individual.

WORTH REPEATING

This bolting of food gives rise to a whole host of problems, such as ulcers, irritable bowel, heartburn, abdominal and intestinal discomfort. In many cases, this is the symptom of a much greater affliction: not knowing how to care for the self.

The mouth

When food is in the mouth, it is tasted, ground down and then mixed with saliva and mucus to aid passage down the throat to the stomach. In a negative eating strategy, the food is chewed enough to fit down the throat. The food is not appreciated or enjoyed, sometimes barely tasted. The food is not masticated enough, which loads extra work onto the stomach. The taste-buds in the mouth act as sensors indicating how much sugar, salt and fats we are eating. When we bolt our food, our sensors are unaware of how much we are taking in, so we eat too much.

The stomach

When food is bolted, it is not masticated properly and reaches the stomach in a lumpy, pasty consistency. The stomach has a hard time aiding digestion. The acids of the stomach are not soaked up properly, and the person will often suffer heartburn, acid reflux or even ulcers. The stomach signals the brain after twenty minutes of eating to tell the brain how full it is. If we bolt food, we can eat too much inside the twenty-minute zone and find ourselves bloated and uncomfortable. Some clients reported the healing and ease of ulcers when processing their food correctly. Food will only leave the stomach comfortably if it is broken down to between one and two millimetres across; otherwise it must be shunted out by the body's house-cleaning operations.

The small intestine

The intestine is packed with food that is not chewed properly or broken down by the stomach. This can give rise to all sorts of intestinal problems as bacteria and gases build up in the system.

The large intestine

When the food is not properly broken down in the mouth, it is not digested correctly in the stomach nor processed evenly in the small intestine. Therefore, by the time it reaches the large intestine, the consistency can be in the extreme. Either it is too gassy and loose or it is too hard. In most cases, bolting food can lead to irritable bowel. Some of my clients suffered from constipation and others from loose, frequent movements. When they began to chew their food well, their symptoms disappeared. This is the likely result of proper processing of food combined with the effects of relaxation and stress release that accompany sensible eating.

The brain

The effect of fast eating on the brain and emotions is, to say the least, counterproductive. Fast eating stresses the body, which inhibits the release of endorphins. Fast eating is damaging for the self-esteem; it is a form of lack of respect for the self. Eating is an important form of self-nurturing; throwing food into the body, with the minimal amount of processing, stresses the entire system. The de-stressing element of eating is lost and the person loses out on the event, while the body becomes more stressed. The brain is compelled to gain satisfaction, so it continues to make the person eat even when full. Satisfaction never comes and the person does not stop eating. When we eat food too fast, the brain cannot discern how much food is being put into the system

---

WE ARE BORN TO CHEW.

Did you ever feed a young child, especially one that has not yet acquired all its teeth? This is definitely something that you cannot rush because the child won't let you. You sit down beside one of those marvels of creation in the high chair, and before you is a plate of mashed food. You take up the spoon and feed it to the baby; the baby accepts it and then, much to your amazement, begins to chew the food. This is part of the child's nature.

My little niece, then five years old, was eating fast food chips and chicken nuggets. She heard her two older brothers coming down the corridor to the kitchen. Mindful that she might have to part with one of her two nuggets from trickery, persuasion or force, she put both of them into her mouth. Her brothers came in, looked at her plate and, seeing no chicken nuggets, went off. "That's a lot of food in there," I said to her and she looked up at me smiled and then nodded a yes. She looked like a hamster whose cheeks were stuffed with golf balls. As I talked to her dad, I secretly counted the amount of chewing she did before she started to swallow. Much to my amazement, she chewed her food eighty times before she began to swallow.

After she had finished swallowing, she left the rest behind and went out to play. Children have this ability built in, unless we teach them otherwise. Unfortunately there are time constraints in modern living. Around the time they reach school-going age, we get our kids up with just enough time to wash, dress and stuff in breakfast; this is when the rot sets in. We force them to start eating fast, not realising how we are compromising them in later life.

We often hear parents saying, "No, you can't have an ice cream; the last time you had one, you did not finish it off and it was a waste." Here the child just ate enough ice cream and tossed the rest because he/she was satisfied. If our children are eating too fast, from whom are they getting this habit? Us. The child obesity in our society is caused by lack of chewing. Teach the children to chew and they will automatically go towards healthy food. The way we teach children is—that's right—by example.

Children chew automatically unless they have learned to bolt their food. This is what is encoded in the child's DNA: "Mix your food with a lot of saliva and enjoy the taste and textures." A child will let you know in no uncertain terms that he/she has had enough. The child's body knows when it is full; they may call for food later on, but now they are satisfied and that's that. This is the way our systems are designed—we do not really have to think about it too much.

A short word about food (the content)

At this stage you might be wondering why I am not really saying anything about what kind of foods to eat and what not to eat. This is because our body knows what to eat. We know how to distinguish the good food from the unhealthy food; the mouth and nose and eyes can guide us: all we have to do is listen to our bodies' sensitivity. It's there—you know it is—it is always telling you, and all you have to do is start listening. If I go down the street and ask people what is healthy food, and what is unhealthy food, they will tell me. Unhealthy food includes foods with too much fat and sugar, like processed meats and confectionery; healthy foods are fresh vegetables, grains, fruits, non-processed dairy and meat. We know what is good for us.

Our bodies are designed to eat from the environment. The variety of foods in their natural state is good for us and for our systems. In many foods there are parts that get rid of toxins in the body. Other foods help clean the blood. There are foods that clean up free radicals, which can cause disease. Most of these foods taken in their natural state have a good balance. But what do we do? Of course, we process them. This has a negative effect on the food-stuff, often cutting out the beneficial parts of the food. For example, we harvest a grain, get rid of the bran, which cleans the system, and grind it down, bleach it, denature it and then make bread and confectionery. When we eat the stuff, it is very difficult to digest and causes extra mucus to be produced in the body. The strange thing is that some of us consider this normal food.

We now eat bulky, saturated food. We have cut out roughage, the very stuff that cleans the system. Food-stuffs like husk, bran, some skins and seed coats have been cut out of our diets. We need a certain amount of roughage to clear the system. If we eat good, fresh food, we feel good and fresh; and if we eat stodgy, highly processed food we feel stodgy and highly processed—that is, stressed.

Some foods are light and some foods are saturated. Saturated foods are full of fat, sugar, dairy products and white flour. Saturated foods have a lot more fat, processed sugar, and processed wheat in them than natural food, such as vegetables, natural grains, organic

71

meat or fruits. When we chew our foods well, and taste the tastes, we become conscious of the quality of foods we take in. The reason why some of us eat too many saturated foods is because we eat them fast. In this way, we have no idea how saturated they are.

A spicy wedge is a deep-fat-fried chunk of potato with a crust of salt and spices on the outside. This is quite tasty and we could probably eat quite a few, if we eat fast without awareness. When we become aware, chew our food well and taste it completely, we find we only need a little to experience satisfaction. By chewing thoroughly and tasting our food, we find ourselves eating fewer and fewer saturated foods, because the taste and feeling of these foods become less appealing. The mouth has taste-buds that react to fatty substances and signal to the brain, which tells the system how much it needs. After a while we don't want any more of the high-saturated food because the brain tells us we've had enough.

WORTH REPEATING

By chewing thoroughly and tasting our food, we find ourselves eating fewer and fewer saturated foods, because the taste and feeling of these foods become less appealing.

By eating naturally, chewing well, tasting and being here, now, while we eat, we don't have to worry about the fatty foods, because we will automatically eat less of them. Choose organic foods—they are better quality. They are more expensive but now we won't be eating too much, and a little will go farther. This way, we do our bit for the environment, creating more environmentally friendly organic farms. We do our bit for the economy by going for local produce. We look after our bodies by eating fresh, natural foods.

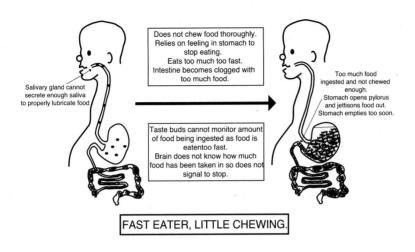

Does not chew food thoroughly.
Relies on feeling in stomach to stop eating.
Eats too much too fast.
Intestine becomes clogged with too much food.

Salivary gland cannot secrete enough saliva to properly lubricate food

Too much food ingested and not chewed enough.
Stomach opens pylorus and jettisons food out.
Stomach empties too soon.

Taste buds cannot monitor amount of food being ingested as food is eatentoo fast.
Brain does not know how much food has been taken in so does not signal to stop.

FAST EATER, LITTLE CHEWING.

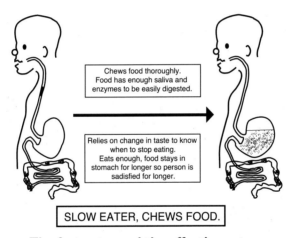

Chews food thoroughly.
Food has enough saliva and enzymes to be easily digested.

Relies on change in taste to know when to stop eating.
Eats enough, food stays in stomach for longer so person is sadisfied for longer.

SLOW EATER, CHEWS FOOD.

The fast eater and the effective eater.

What if I choose not to chew my food thoroughly?

1. I will continue to eat too much.
2. I will continue to eat the wrong foods.
3. I will not reach my ideal slimness.
4. I am choosing to damage my digestive system.

5. I am choosing not to love myself.
6. I am choosing low confidence and self-esteem.
7. I am choosing to make eating a misery.

What if I choose to chew my food thoroughly?

1. I will eat the right amount of food.
2. I will enjoy the right foods.
3. I will slim automatically.
4. I am choosing a healthy digestive system.
5. I am choosing to love myself.
6. I choose high confidence and self-esteem.
7. I am choosing to make eating a pleasure.

Conclusion

Eating our food too fast or not masticating it properly can come from the stresses and strains of a time-limited modern lifestyle. We may have lost a lot of the sensitivity we need to nurture our body and mind correctly. However, putting an unhealthy eating routine before health is asking for trouble, unless you want to be miserable, unhealthy and stressed.

Begin by practising chewing food forty times a mouthful. Be in the here and now; when the taste of the food becomes a little less pleasurable, stop. Eat whatever you desire; just chew well to let your taste-buds monitor your intake.

Eating too fast = Misery, unhealthiness and stress.
Eating sensibly = Happiness, health and love.

The choice is yours . . .

Part III

The Importance of Movement

Chapter 5

Movement for Your Mind: The emotional and mental benefits of movement

---

Body movement is play—enjoy it. A tremendous amount of joy and happiness can be experienced through a little body movement.

In this chapter I often use the term *movement*, because any movement is exercise. We tend, however, to see exercise as something we do in a gym or with a machine or in a class. In fact, dancing is exercise—as are gardening, housework, washing the car, painting a wall, putting boxes in the attic, pushing a lawn mower, cycling, and many other everyday activities.

We need to move; we are built for it. We are large predators, built to roam over long distances hunting and gathering every day. We still have the same bodies our ancestors had twenty thousand years ago. Human beings are good walkers; we can walk other animals into the ground; we are physically powerful. Not moving such a powerful body, not giving it exercise, is asking for trouble.

How do we destroy motivation for exercise? Simple—by exercising to lose weight. We need to exercise for joy, fun, health and to clean the body. Exercising to lose weight is too much of a long-term goal. Losing weight, as you know now, is a low value, and it is difficult to motivate oneself for a low value. So many people look at exercise as a chore rather than a means to clean the body, induce a positive, resourceful mood and increase intelligence and social interaction.

Chapter overview

Why we fail to exercise

We tend to give up when
1. exercising to become slim
2. exercising becomes a punishment

How to succeed

Engage in movement for
1. emotional stability
2. increased intelligence
3. social interaction

Do not exercise to become slim; exercise to *feel good*. Increase your desire to exercise; make the time; enjoy your exercise. At the start work up to walk or move briskly for forty minutes once a day and that is enough. Get a bicycle and cycle. Breathe deeply for a couple of breaths every now and again. Choose pleasant surroundings and pleasant people to exercise with; you will live longer with a better quality of life and better feelings—if you don't, you won't. The body and mind need exercise. There are six powerful reasons to exercise and none of them have to do with losing weight. In this chapter we will look at the first three reasons to exercise, and in the next chapter, the remaining three.

Why we fail to exercise

So what stops us from doing our exercise? What could be so difficult about going out for a walk and burning all the calories off? After all, even if we ate too much food but exercised a lot, we would be slim. What happens to our motivation—why do we find simple movement so difficult? Often the reason is that we start exercising to become slim, rather than exercising for its own sake. We exercise to punish ourselves for eating too much or for being overweight.

1. Exercising to become slim

When we exercise to become slim, our motivation is weakly supported by a goal that is usually too far away. If I am trying to lose weight and I do some hard exercise, I will not find much has changed when I jump on the scales. If I am driving myself with negativity, this will certainly not put myself in favour after all my hard work. This leads to discouragement. I am working at exercising to get slim and to get away from my self-criticism, but when I stand on the scales again, there is little change and the self-criticism gets worse. Now the thought of exercise is painful, so I avoid it. I feel bad for not doing it but feel worse when I try. "I am fat and no good and should be ashamed of my body"; "I have no control and I eat too much"—these are the criticisms I heap on myself. I do anything to avoid exercise because there is nothing but negativity surrounding it. Exercising to become slim usually does not work. We need to focus on the good feelings that exercising produces, and exercise for its own sake.

2. Exercise becomes a punishment

When we are exercising to punish ourselves, we usually choose painful exercises or choose ones that are hard to do. "Now I must go to the gym and burn the lard off" kind of stuff. In this frame of mind, and after a long day's work, we must get into the car, drive to the gym, dress in our gear, and sweat and groan our way through an exercise regime or a jogging routine. Not only that, but we imagine that all the good-looking, trim-muscled other people will be looking at us with mockery and disdain. Not an easy thing to motivate ourselves for, is it? I think I would rather lie here on the couch and eat chocolate chip cookies. Punishing does not work, and punishing ourselves with exercise corrupts a wonderful, natural pleasure—the pleasure of movement for movement's sake. We need to make the exercise as pleasurable as possible and as easy to do as possible.

Human beings usually avoid pain and seek pleasure. We are willing to put up with a little discomfort if there is immediate pleasure afterwards, but otherwise most of us will avoid discomfort. The secret of enjoying exercise is to experience the good feelings we get from it now.

How to succeed

Everything that is good for our survival has pleasure associated with it. Eating, exercise and sex—if we did not enjoy any of these activities, we would be extinct by now. For we might never have engaged in them often enough to secure our survival.

Just using the eating strategy alone reduces weight; most of the time that is all one has to do. It usually leads, however, to people wanting to exercise because they feel much better about themselves and have more energy. The best way is to exercise when you feel like it—do not force yourself. It typically happens that people begin exercise because, as they feel lighter, they go for the sheer joy of moving their lighter bodies. Do not exercise to slim; exercise to feel good.

There are at least five beneficial effects of proper eating: self-nurturing, emotional well-being, psychological well-being, de-stressing and socialising. Several very important benefits also result from exercising, and these are:

1. Emotional stability

Just as the body benefits from a natural eating strategy so, too, it gains from exercising. Endorphins are released during eating, and dopamine is realised during exercising. Dopamine is important for feeling good and we need a dose of endorphins a day to keep us in good mental and physical health. Dopamine is an interesting hormone because it is also one of the chemicals that are released when we are in love.

It is common knowledge that exercise can alleviate depression. Essentially, it releases dopamine into the system, which picks the person up and improves their mood. When the mood is improved, the person usually finds a way out of the depression.

FACT

A team of German researchers studied twelve people with severe depression that had lasted an average of nine months. In ten of these patients, drugs had failed to bring about any substantial improvement. The group was put through an exercise program that involved walking on a treadmill every day for thirty minutes. Three minutes of intensive activity was alternated with walking at half speed for three minutes. The researchers at Freie University of Berlin found that, after ten days, six patients were "substantially less depressed", including five that had not been helped by drugs; two were less depressed while four others were less noticeably changed. (*The Irish Times*, March 2000)

As you can see, the above results were after only ten days, with severely depressed people. Imagine what exercise could do for us if we brought it into our daily routine. Exercise and body movement are adult play. Another very good reason for exercise is that it bonds us socially. The bond we feel when we are engaging with others in the same activities is strong—just as when we are eating with somebody. We tend to make better bonds with people with whom we do things rather than with those who do not share our pastimes. Because body movement brings good feelings, it is an excellent way to meet people while enjoying a physical activity together.

2. Increased intelligence

The body and mind are one system. The amount of nutrients and oxygen getting to the brain is essential for our ability to use the brain. Scientists are now experimenting with fitness to increase mental capacity. The brain is like a large muscle: The more we use the brain cells, the thicker they get. The thicker they get, the more oxygen and nutrients they need to run them and the more blood they need to nourish them.

When our bodies engage in exercise, they become oxygenated; the blood runs freely through the system carrying more oxygen and nutrients to the brain. This increases our ability to concentrate and use our minds. Exercise produces chemicals that affect the hypocampus and causes it to produce more brain cells. Essentially, exercise increases intelligence. Scientists are noticing the beneficial effects of exercise on the brain. The proverbial high-achiever who is both captain of the school team and top of the class is a self-fulfilling prophesy. New studies on the brain are influencing the introduction of more exercise into school systems to increase successful results. These schools will see higher performance academically, and not only that, but the students will be more emotionally and socially stable.

Get the edge, clear your mind and increase its capacity and speed; exercise for increasing your own intelligence. Exercise is one of the most underestimated beneficial activities, and one of the most easy to do. Start off with a very simple exercise like walking. The most important thing is to develop the habit. Walk for five minutes out the road, turn and walk back. Every two days or so, increase the time by another five minutes. Walk in beautiful areas, places that you like. Cycling is another good activity to do—easy and economical.

CASE HISTORY

One day, in through my office door came a woman who was very overweight. I told her that if she were too overweight, I would not work with her because of safety. She would have to get medical attention. She assured me that she was several stone overweight but not as heavy as she looked.

She had a part-time job in an office and, after work, mostly sat and watched television in her flat. That was about it as regards her activity. While watching TV, she ate extraordinary amounts of food as well as her three to six meals a day, all mostly saturated fats.

I explained about how to chew her food thoroughly and taste each morsel. We talked about chewing her food up to forty times or more a mouthful, and how the body needs to swallow only fine soup. I explained how this realisation and action would get her natural sensitivity back again to eat just what she needs.

The next session she came in and told me how she was only eating a third of what she normally consumed. She was amazed at how easy it was and expressed a desire to do exercise to help her slimming along, but she did not like exercising. I introduced her to the idea of exercise for the sake of exercising, not for slimming. I also explained how moving the body gives us a natural high and we can be more effective in life when we exercise.

Because of her weight, walking was the only exercise available to her, but she was very self-conscious about how she looked and felt embarrassed in public. She mentioned that she liked music so I suggested that she get a set of headphones and walk with her favourite music. I suggested just ten minutes a day, to be built up to half an hour in a week's time. In the next session, despite my advice to start gently at ten minutes, she reported that she was now walking several miles every day and really enjoying it.

The next time she came in I could see the difference, and that is when she confessed that she had not told me the truth about her weight; she was actually two stone heavier than she'd said. She explained that she was afraid that I would not take her on if I knew her weight. I saw her every second week just for ten minutes or so. Each time she came in, she was far lighter than before, shedding nearly a half stone a week. I was concerned about her rapid weight loss, but she assured me she was having a great time. It was amazing to see her change—like watching a sculpture walk out of a block of marble.

> The only changes she really made were to enjoy
> her food for food's sake and enjoy her exercise
> for itself. Essentially, she took her focus off being
> overweight and directed it to quality of life. Her
> natural ability to enjoy herself did the rest. If we feel
> good about ourselves, we find it easier to do things
> we want to do.

3. Social interaction

You might already recognise my point here: Not only do people eat to socialise, but they also do activities to socialise. One of the biggest problems on the planet is loneliness. A lot of people exercise for socialising: " I joined the tennis club to get fit and get to know people in my neighbourhood." When people embark on this sort of programme, they often change in many ways for the better. Several of my clients have reported new social connections because of taking up an activity.

Socialising can be a strain when done in circumstances where there is nothing else going on. Imagine going into a place and sitting opposite a stranger and starting cold: "Hello, my name is . . ." It is much easier if we are doing something together, an activity through which we can relate. We can find out more about others by simply watching and listening to them and then deciding if we want to get to know them better or not.

Conclusion

Move the body to enjoy life. Figure out the way you enjoy moving your body, whether this be dancing, walking, swimming or other activity. Then do it often, exercise to enhance health, happiness, and life—and for no other reason. We strive in life to succeed in order to be happy. Sometimes it is better to find out what it is that makes us happy, and do a bit more of it. Things like eating and exercising are good for our happiness and we are happy doing them as well—talk about a win-win situation!

Exercise to:

1. Feel good. The body produces hormones when we exercise and these hormones give us a natural high. When we exercise, we feel good; we become emotionally stronger and better able to handle life's ups and downs.

2. Increase intelligence. During exercise the body produces chemicals that increase the production of brain cells. By exercising we open up the body's respiratory system, increase the efficiency of both uptake in vitamins and the secretion of waste products. More oxygen is available for the brain to think—essentially: healthy body, healthy mind.

3. Enjoy social interaction. Doing activities with other people is a very good way of enjoying ourselves. Going for a walk with another person, cycling, attending yoga class, playing football or practicing martial arts are among the many activities that will expand your circle of friends and enhance your quality of life.

Chapter 6

Movement for Your Body: The physical benefits of movement

We live with and through our bodies; health is a prime value, more important than wealth, being slim or having many "things".

The human being is a top predator; we are large animals, built to hunt over wide areas of land. Our bodies still hold the grace and power of the hunter-gatherer. The average western adult human is heavier than a wolf, a leopard or a hyena. These are big game animals, and so are we. We are built to move; it is part of our nature. Animals are happy doing what they are built for and so are we. Humans need to move, to roam, to exercise.

Chapter overview

1. Movement to clean the body

An enormous amount of the body's waste products is released through the breath. We need to exercise to enhance our breathing to clean the body. Movement aids digestion.

2. Movement for health and happiness

Our muscle tone, bone strength, and the health of our inner organs depend on body movement. Use it or lose it. Health is a top value; by looking after it we promote well-being.

3. Renew emotional, mental and physical state

Movement can be a break from other activities. Exercise is a good way to get out of negative states or to combat work fatigue. It strengthens the mind and body and makes us better at everything else.

1. Movement to clean the body

When exercising, we breathe more deeply than normal, which has a profound effect on increasing health in the body. Breathing is very important, because a large amount of our bodies' waste products are released through our breath. So what is the primary exit of toxins from the body? Yes, it is the breath. When we breath in oxygen, we help burn up calories. When we breathe deeply, we massage our gut which aids peristalsis, the movement of food through the intestine. In this way, deep breathing has a cleansing effect, and the food does not hang around the gut too long; therefore, the system does not over-absorb or toxify. Breathing also runs the lymphatic system; this is the system that cleans the blood. When your diaphragm moves up and down as you inhale and exhale it also pumps the lymph around the body. The lymphatic system does not have a heart; it relies on your breathing to pump it around your body.

When we are exercising, we breathe more deeply than when we are stationary. Breathing is very important for health and energy. Many martial arts masters use breath alone for developing real power.

Breathing exercises add many years of quality to our lives. It is handy to experiment with breathing when exercising, or even when sitting or standing. To clean the body, breathe in deeply, hold the breath for a second and then let it out long and slow. This is good for cleaning the body and releasing stress.

It is believed that quite a lot of cellulite, the fatty tissue that is soft and lumpy in appearance, stores toxins that we intake from food. Breathing is a very successful way to clean the body and oxygenate the system for health and fitness. If we become overweight, sometimes we reduce the capacity of our lungs, thus getting less oxygen and therefore eliminating fewer toxins from our bodies.

Exercise causes us to breathe more rapidly and more deeply, and this

1. cleans waste products and toxins from the body;
2. supplies oxygen to burn up more calories;
3. aids peristalsis, moving food efficiently through the gut;
4. pumps lymph around the body, which cleans the blood.

2. Movement for health and happiness

Happiness is a skill of living, and moving the body is part of that skill. Exercise to increase happiness; do we need any other reason? Human beings are meant to be fit—that is our natural state. Some bodies have the capacity to be fitter than others, but all are built to be fit. If we are fit, we recover from illness faster, break down food more efficiently and even think better. The systems of the body work normally if we are fit; they do not work well if we are unfit. When we are unfit and do not move around, we start to build up excess energy in the body, clogging our system. But when we move our bodies, this requires energy; therefore, the more we move and exercise, the more we use up energy and the lighter we get. Fat is excess energy. We do not, however, have to go to the gym and exert ourselves with painful exercises to be happy. Human beings are good walkers, and walking is often enough exercise to promote well-being.

Health is a high value, and when we are supporting a high value, it builds our self-esteem. Many of us have heard the phrase "your health is your wealth"; certainly, when we are ill, nothing else seems to matter more than to get back to good health. For most people health is a top value and usually (but not always) takes second or third place below happiness. Fun is a related and frequently underestimated value: When people are exercising, they are more inclined to laugh and release stress.

It takes as much energy to briskly walk a mile/kilometre as it does to run a mile/kilometre. The only difference, of course, is the time factor. It is interesting to think that with every step we take when we are walking, we are by increments getting lighter.

3. Renew emotional, mental and physical state

Exercise is a great way to break out of, or enhance, a particular state of being. By *state of being* I mean the mental, emotional and physical feelings we have at any one time. We can experience states of happiness, sadness, frustration, boredom, humour, fatigue and so on. If we are in a state of sadness, boredom or stress, doing exercise can break us out of that state into a positive state. Often people complain about being too tired or too stressed to do anything. The best way to get energy is to use it; you get back what you put out. It is so easy to come home after a long day at work and say, "I'm too tired to do anything." We can easily break the state of fatigue by just going for a short walk, getting outside and bringing the mind into the here and now.

How much movement should we do? Studies vary, but if we gave five hours of vigorous exercise a week, we would not be getting it wrong. Some people consider five hours to be a lot and others feel it's not enough. Either way, the benefits of movement far outweigh the reasons for not getting any exercise. There are an average of sixteen waking hours in a day, which is one hundred and twelve hours in a week. As we can see, we have time.

CASE HISTORY

I was working with a man who was slightly overweight and had a very stressful job. The focus of the sessions was on stress. He had mentioned the weight as something he would like to address in the future. When I introduced the idea of exercise, he said simply, "I don't have the time; I'm too busy." "Exactly," I said. "If you don't have time to exercise, you are *too* busy." His life was a typical example of the lives of many people who suffer from stress and being overweight. The fundamental issue is: no variety in life.

He had work, and he had little rest and no play. Work, sleep; work, sleep; work, sleep; death. The only reason he was resting was because he had to go home to sleep. When he needed to fuel himself, he ate fast, standing up, while he consumed rich, saturated convenience foods. He admitted he was short tempered with his family and that they never appreciated all the work he was doing for them. His experience was typical of that of a lot of men: They go to work longer hours to provide more for their families; but families "want their presence not their presents". They give things in the expression of love, but we know people love us when they cannot help being in our presence.

At work, his boss was onto him about his efficiency so, of course, he tried to work even harder, taking more time away from his family. I persuaded him that he needed a break from his home and work, something that he could do that was easy. He agreed to park his car about two miles away from his office and walk. That is four miles a day. At first he found it a nuisance as he adjusted to earlier times going to work and later times coming home. My thinking behind this was threefold: one—to get him to take some time alone so he could think; two—to increase the good chemical dopamine in his system, released by the exercise; and three—to increase his good health and reduce stress.

In his third session he reported feeling better; his thinking was much clearer and he decided to come home earlier in the evenings. He was amazed to discover that spending less time at work actually made him more efficient. Then we focused on chewing, which caused him to sit with his family longer at the table, which in turn strengthened his bond with them. His family was now feeling cared for and responded positively to his presence. Introducing body movement into our lives has huge benefits: It allows us to do everything else even better.

What if you don't move your body?

1. My moods are less positive.
2. My confidence is low.
3. My mind is not as quick.
4. My body becomes more toxic.
5. I am less healthy and get sick more often.

6. Everything else is unlikely to improve.
7. I continue to live with diminished quality of life.

What if you move your body?

1. I feel increasingly better and better.
2. My confidence overall becomes stronger.
3. My mind becomes more intelligent.
4. My body becomes more cleansed of toxins.
5. I become healthier and get fewer ailments.
6. Everything else in my life improves.
7. I enjoy good quality of life.

Conclusion

Our bodies are our minds. The nervous system is concentrated in the skull cavity, but it is spread throughout the body. By keeping the body fit, we benefit everything else. Human beings need variety; exercise provides the kind of variety that can change state of mind. Humans are happy when they are moving—what better reason to walk, dance, play sports, be active and get fit?

Chapter 7

A Case History

Pleasure is part of happiness and happiness is part of contentment.

Let us look again at the three major areas where we run into trouble as we try to shed weight. The first is our attitude; the second is the way we process food; and the third is exercise or body movement. If we have a negative attitude, we will get negative results. If we do not eat our food according to the way the body is designed, we will eat too much. If we use exercise to lose weight, it can become a punishment and we won't do it.

Chapter overview

Below is a case history that I call 'the milk-chocolate eater'. It provides a typical example of what we can experience when we use negativity. It shows how the sin-guilt-punishment-damnation cycle begins—and how it ends.

The milk-chocolate eater

CASE HISTORY

A woman came into my consulting rooms with a problem, and the problem was eating chocolate. She said that every night, without fail, she would eat two or three bars of chocolate, and that this had contributed to her gaining weight.

"So what's the problem?" I asked. "Don't you enjoy the chocolate more than you enjoy being slim?"

"No," she said emphatically, "I hate myself for eating the chocolate, but I can't stop. I should be exercising every day, but I don't; my body is horribly fat and disgusting, and I am so miserable. If only I was slim, everything would be wonderful." Then she started crying.

I was delighted because I knew exactly what she was doing and exactly the solutions to her problem. "Your problem is not the slimming," I said. "It is the negative thoughts and self-put-downs that are making you feel so bad."

What is it that keeps her eating the chocolate, even though she dislikes herself for doing so? How does one eat that amount of chocolate without getting fed up or sick? Simple: We have to throw the chocolate into the body quickly, and we have to do it with the least amount of awareness—in other words, by being "not there". The only way to eat three big bars of chocolate is by disregarding the self and eating fast, very fast.

So how did she eat two or three bars of chocolate a night? Again, the answer is simple: by disliking herself for doing so. I asked, "Tell me how you eat that much chocolate; if I could eat that much chocolate a night and enjoy it, I would be a happy man."

She sighed, looked down and began her story. "I get up in the morning and I start dieting because I have eaten chocolate the night before. I am totally disgusted with myself."

The story was what I expected. She went on to tell me she ate an apple and black tea for breakfast, a glass of water for break, a banana and yoghurt for lunch, and boiled chicken and broccoli for tea. She continues to punish herself and so feels more and more miserable; a slimming life has little to offer except months of misery, diets and negative put-downs for the future. Then her motivation and will break under the strain and, a little later, she goes out and buys her first chocolate bar. Then she goes out and buys a second and sometimes a third. Of course she eats the lot. She gives up, and the next day, in a state of misery and guilt, eats everything around her. She beats herself up all day under the illusion that negativity will motivate her not to eat. Then she plans an eat-nothing diet and a visit to the gym, where she intends to do a hundred reps on every machine but, of course, she never does. One of the practical issues here is her blood sugar; by the evening her blood sugar would be very low and she would not have the energy to do very much anyway. This is how attitude sets up the sin-guilt-punishment-damnation cycle.

The sin-guilt-punishment-damnation cycle

The Sin

To sin is just missing the mark—it's normal and natural to make mistakes. Mistakes are feedback mechanisms that give us learning and knowledge. Problems arise when we look at missing the mark as a failure of our person. Mary continued to describe herself as "bad" the day after eating too much chocolate the night before. "I ate too much chocolate; therefore I am a bad person." And "I did not exercise, so I am a big fat slob." Remember the story of the picture of the cat. Negativity, when taken personally, destroys motivation.

The Guilt

Guilt is just the compulsion to try again; there is nothing wrong with it unless it is done negatively. Mary vows never to eat chocolate again. In the morning her conviction is very strong. She puts herself down for hours on end: " I'm bad, I have no will, I'm disgusting, my body is horrible." Negative guilt sets us up for failure because the weight of negativity causes too much punishment.

She vows to eat practically nothing and exercise herself into the ground.

The Punishment

Punishment is just limitation if it is used appropriately; in the positive sense, it is a skill builder. When we use it to make us feel bad, however, it destroys our will, motivation and self-esteem. Mary starts dieting. All day long she puts herself down, wearing away her will, motivation and self-esteem. All day long she thinks of "not food", which is programming herself to eat while, at the same time, she is stopping herself from eating. She limits her good feelings and does not allow herself to feel good, happy or satisfied until she has done an hour and a half of exercise and eaten minimally. Even then, all her good feelings are being put off until she meets her goal of being slim, which would be in several months time. Looking forward to several months of misery breaks any person's will, especially when the goal is a low value.

Damnation

Damnation happens when we make negative judgements about ourselves. Mary feels so wretched that she gives up and then buys and eats too much chocolate. Damnation attacks the sense of self and lowers self-esteem. The next day the whole thing starts again. Eating a few bars of chocolate is not something to damage our self-esteem—our health maybe—but not our self-esteem. With damnation, the punishment does not fit the crime—it is too severe. Mary's problem is not the eating of the chocolate but the negative self-put-downs.

How did we sort out the problem? Simple—we got Mary to enjoy her chocolate. It took some persuading to get her to agree to eat a little chocolate with me in the office. I explained that chocolate was a special treat and not to be wolfed down. After all, when we eat too fast only a small amount of a square of chocolate touches our taste-buds, the rest might as well be river mud. So we began with the chocolate-eating session. The way to eat chocolate, or any other food for that matter, is roughly in three stages.

The three stages of enjoying food:

(i) *Positive anticipation.* In the anticipation or appreciation stage, thank the universe for what you are about to receive. We sat down with the chocolate and brought our attention into the here and now. We enjoyed the anticipation of eating the chocolate. It's important to use the sense of smell here. As much as possible, smell your food as a way of appreciating before you eat.

(ii) *Positive acceptance*. Then we placed the chocolate into our mouths and sat back and revelled in the taste. In this stage it's important to focus on enjoying the taste and texture, and to taste as much of the chocolate as possible before swallowing it. It is no good just to chew and swallow and gulp more down. We don't use up a whole bottle of shampoo just to wash our hair once, because it is unnecessary.

(iii) *Positive appreciation*. The third stage is enjoying the feeling after eating. When we finished the chocolate, we spent time thinking about how nice it was and what an enjoyable way to pass a few minutes—thanking the universe for the pleasure we had shared. After I had gotten Mary to eat a little chocolate in this way, I pointed to the clock. We had been enjoying two squares of chocolate for fifteen minutes.

We had some more chocolate—guilt free— anticipating, tasting, feeling and then reminiscing. Mary was delighted to reach the stage of satisfaction, where she'd had enough and to eat more would spoil the enjoyment. All things lose their pleasure when we do them too much and for too long. I asked her not to exercise at all because I wanted her to be as guilt free as possible for now. Part of the agreement was that she would buy three big bars of milk chocolate now, before she went home, and look forward to enjoying as much as she might want that evening. She agreed that the next day she would try positive self-talk and eat a healthy breakfast, lunch and tea, with nibbles at break times. She said that she doubted that such a positive approach would work, but she was willing to give it a try. She left the office with a backward glance that could have been mistaken as doubt of my sanity.

Four days later, I got the phone call from a very happy, satisfied chocolate eater. She was down to a half bar in the evening time. Her self-esteem was getting better, because she was now nurturing, not punishing, herself. Her next session focused on exercise. She was trying exercising to lose weight and began to realise that, in her mind, exercise was a punishment. Going to the gym seemed like such a big chore. I found out that she liked walking and swimming. So the next step was to get her to walk a little every day and walk only for the feel-good chemicals and the fresh air. She felt that it was a time constraint to drive out to the park and do a walk and then drive back. She came up with the idea to park her car thirty minutes away from her work where the parking was cheaper and more convenient to her homeward journey.

She reported in the next session that she enjoyed the walking and reached work in the morning and home in the evening in a fresher, more positive mood. She is also doing her bit for the environment. The third session she came in and was upset because she had eaten a whole bar of chocolate the night before. During the week, once or twice, she drove to work and did not walk. I explained to her that it is important that we factor in times when things don't go as planned. The most important action to take is not to cut ourselves down negatively if we do not do what we had originally intended.

If we miss the mark, there are three things we need to do:

(1) focus on what we can do better next time;

(2) focus on the good things we are doing;

(3) focus on practising positively in the future.

Mary explored how this was the first time since her childhood that she had ever eaten in such a balanced way and felt good. This was the first time she actually enjoyed exercise since she was a child. She reported that before she had eaten the whole bar of chocolate, she had not felt good. She could see that, next time, doing something to directly address the feeling would be a better strategy than overeating. When she drove to work, she was feeling tired after watching a late movie the night before. She realised she felt even more tired without her walk and the next time she could do it in the evening. It is important to expect that the odd day things will not go as planned. She then set out a few pointers for the future in order to exercise to feel good and to do things she likes to balance her emotions.

The next session, she reported that her clothes were loosening and she was shedding weight. She had missed her walk again one day and had gone to the gym instead and really enjoyed it. She said her chewing was automatic now, and she was eating less food with more satisfaction. Like others, she found that the most important change is the freedom from negativity. When she eats a little too much, or misses her walk the odd day, she does not beat herself up, causing loss of motivation. She just resolves to get back on track next time.

What kind of magic happened? Eating the chocolate in the office, while being in the here and now, helped train her in the art of sensitivity and guilt-free pleasure. It was important to let her give herself permission to enjoy the chocolate. By realising the pleasure in chocolate, we actually eat less. The sensation and taste of the chocolate on the taste-buds are what is giving the pleasure here and now. Swallowing that chocolate and putting more in is a waste of time, because we do not have taste-buds in our stomachs. Eating loads of chocolate is comparable to buying your favourite music, listening to it for a while, stopping it before the end of the track, then going out, buying it again and starting all over. Buying ten copies of a favourite album will not help us enjoy it more. You end up sick of the music, broke and dissatisfied.

If we really enjoy food, why do we eat so much that we feel bad? That is not enjoying food. If we like exercise, we don't continue exercising for twelve steady hours and still enjoy it, do we? If we enjoy watching TV, would we still be entertained after watching twenty-four hours non-stop? If your passion were golf, would you still be as enthusiastic after 280 holes of solid play? Overdoing it is not the way you enjoy golf, TV, or exercise—and it certainly is not the way to enjoy food.

By giving herself permission to eat, Mary released
the struggle of "I can. I can't"—no struggle, no war,
no loss, no pain. Choosing positive self-talk increased
motivation and self-liking. Eating breakfast and lunch
stopped the massive build-up of hunger and tamed
the reptilian brain. Knowing that she can still have her
chocolate, and have full permission to eat it and enjoy
it, stopped the obsession. It became less important and
blended into the other things she enjoys throughout
her day. Doing her exercise became a pleasure that
enhanced everything else.

She reached her ideal slim figure and had the quality of
life and the positive mind-set to enjoy it.

Conclusion

Negativity does not work; self-put-downs, from sin to damnation, only destroy motivation and self-esteem. Negativity stresses the body and reduces energy; it is unhealthy. If we want to succeed, we need to use *towards* attitudes, focusing on well-being and happiness.

Eating affects the mental, physical and emotional parts of the self. All these parts are involved when we eat. Each part exacts an amount of satisfaction from eating food. Food should be enjoyed—it is one of the pleasures of life. When people start to negatively deny themselves food, the trouble begins. If you fall out with food, food becomes a problem.

The secret to an ideal eating strategy is to like your food and to enjoy it as much as possible. Most people who want to slim say,

"That's the problem—I like my food too much." But eating too much and eating too fast are definitely not enjoying food. We like a hot bath—it is lovely and relaxing—but would we therefore like a boiling bath even more? Overeating is not enjoying food; it's a form of force-feeding. It is more difficult to eat greater amounts of food than smaller amounts. Stop using yourself as a compost bin. In other words, by enjoying our food more, do we eat less? Yes.

We need to let our bodies decide how much they want by giving our taste-buds time to monitor the amounts of food we eat. Our bodies have highly sophisticated equipment for monitoring the amounts of sugars, fats, salts, proteins and starches that enter the system. They cannot work if we wolf our food down; we need to chew our food for our bodies to monitor the intake.

Do not exercise to slim; exercise for the good feelings exercise brings. Exercise is movement, not pain; choose exercise that you enjoy and that you can do conveniently and easily at the start. In this way, we look forward to movement, instead of finding it easy to avoid. Movement is play; play releases stress and supports happiness.

Part IV

Developing the Three Happy Habits of Sensual Slimming

Chapter 8

The Happy Habit of a Positive Attitude

The art of happiness is not such that it is bound to big events, successes or revelations. Rather, it is the small innocent things like a nice meal, a good walk, an amiable conversation with an acquaintance or friend, the smile of a child, or just observing the innocent thoughts and words of goodness.

Before I knew how to eat, I always used to be amazed when someone would be given a chocolate bar, eat it slowly and then leave the rest till later. I could not understand the concept; if I had a chocolate bar, I would eat it regardless of whether I was full or not. Over the years, I have come to understand the strategy that these people automatically use: They live in the now. They are positive toward people. They allow their bodies to tell them how much to eat, and when.

Chapter overview

The happy habit of a positive attitude

Let's look at how to practise the first principle of the sensual slimming strategy, a positive attitude, which involves:

1. The thinking behind a positive attitude. Open versus closed thinking.

2. The language behind a positive attitude. What words to use and how to use them.

3. The imagery behind a positive attitude. What pictures to use and how to use them.

4. The feelings behind a positive attitude. What feelings to use and how to use them.

Overall, the idea is to increase quality of life and be happier—now.

The happy habit of a positive attitude

Maintaining a positive attitude when it comes to the matter of weight can be hard for some people, especially with current social conditioning that overweight is not as attractive as healthy weight. However, self-dissatisfaction generates lack of motivation. In my experience, people are more likely to do something when they feel good about themselves. People with good self-esteem generally achieve more than people who have poor self-esteem. Poor self-esteem is made up of self-dislike or non-acceptance of the self. After all, why would you do something for someone you don't like or accept? On the other hand, it's so easy to do something for someone you do accept. If we have extra weight on our bodies and dislike our bodies, this can become generalised into disliking and not accepting ourselves. If we don't like or accept our bodies, we generally find it hard to motivate ourselves for positive change.

One of the things clients really like about the sensual slimming strategy is that just letting go of all the obsessive thoughts and negative self-put-downs about weight is such a joy. Some say that alone is enough. They experience a quality of life straightaway and their newfound, positive, effective thinking leads them to slim. Some people try to implement the eating strategy but they do not give up the negativity. "OK, I will try your strategy, but I am not going to let go of thinking I am a big fat slob." It's as though they are using the negativity to manipulate themselves towards being slim, but this has not worked in the past and will not work in the future. The great thing to remember is that eating is a pleasure from which we can gain a lot of satisfaction; and the more we get into the satisfaction, the more healthy it is for us. The more enjoyment we get from eating, the less we eat. In order to change your attitude, start to programme your mind with positive, rational imagery and thought. Every thought, image, or word that we have in our minds affects us immediately—mentally, emotionally and physically; we are always at prayer. In other words, we cannot have a thought, an image or a word that does not affect us. This is why it is crucial to clear our minds of negative language and imagery while, instead, we use effective language, imagery and thought with positive feeling.

WORTH REPEATING

Every thought, image, or word that we have in our minds affects us immediately—mentally, emotionally and physically; we are always at prayer.

One of the most powerful forms of using your mind positively is increasing your learning or open thinking and using closed or judging thinking in its appropriate place.

1. The thinking behind a positive attitude. Open versus closed thinking.

Now let's again remind ourselves of the three elements of the sensual slimming method. The three elements are: a positive, rational attitude; the process of chewing and enjoying food; and the enjoyment of body movement and exercise. Instead of negative put-downs toward ourselves, we will use positive language and imagery. The best way to think about these three elements is to use open thinking, open thinking is powerful for learning and self motivation. Open thinking and closed thinking in there appropriate contexts produce highly successful results.

Closed thinking is when we think or judge something to be either/or: black or white, good or bad, right or wrong. There is only one way or the other. Either I am fat and ugly or I am slim and perfect. I am either attractive or I am not attractive. I am slimming or I am getting fat. I am "good" if I starve and I am "bad" when I eat. This is yo-yo thinking, which creates a yo-yo attitude and yo-yo diets. It is a win-lose way of thinking. We win when we are starving or sweating in the gym and we lose if we are not. With this way of thinking, we will always lose, because the winning will only be temporary. Closed thinking however is very good for safety issues. If we do not put on our safety belt we get a fine because this is a dangerous way to drive. If we go over the speed limit, we get a fine because it's dangerous to drive fast. If we commit a crime, we get incarcerated because we become a danger to society. These examples illustrate black-and-white, closed thinking and, in such cases, it is good for safety. Using open thinking in a safety situation is disastrous, and most disasters are caused by this process.

Open thinking is good for everything else outside of safety. Open thinking gives us an accurate and open description of our world. Instead of thinking *I am unattractive and ugly,* be practical; an accurate description would be: "I am 12 kg overweight." *Unattractive* and *ugly* are judgements and not accurate, because there is no measure on what is unattractive and ugly. There is no department, no clinic, no international standard to determine what is unattractive and ugly. Beauty is in the eye of the beholder. You may think that you are ugly, but someone who finds you attractive cannot be persuaded otherwise. When we are engaged in closed or judgement thinking, there are typically only two options—black or white. When we are open in our thinking, there are usually several options.

Open thinking or learning thinking. This is good for thinking about relationships, health, career, behaviour, self, and others. Open thinking has distinctive characteristics that will help you recognise and practise it.

1.   Open thinking generates several options instead of just one or two, sometimes expressed in the form of a question.

I would like something sweet; I could have a little chocolate or a cookie. I could eat it slowly, enjoy it more and have a little. Or would I feel more satisfied if I ate an apple?

I look at many options and choices rather than can or cannot have something sweet.

2.   Open thinking increases information by getting the mind to search and consider.

I forgot to go for my walk today. I wonder what kind of reminders I need to put in place for next time so that I can enjoy life much more. *A rational mindset helps me learn from my mistakes and do better next time.*

3.   Open thinking or learning thinking is based on encouragement—win-win.

I am doing well; a couple of times, I did not chew and bolted my food but, more often than not, the habit is getting stronger. I am in the win-win zone. *I constantly encourage myself building stronger motivations.*

4.   Open thinking is based on responsibility, the ability to respond rather than being a victim.

I had lunch with my friend who eats her food fast; I ended up eating mine fast as well but I am responsible for my eating habits. Next time, I am going to enjoy the food much more and maybe introduce her to a new way of enjoying life by savouring the taste of food. *I am responsible for my world and my behaviours.*

5.   Open thinking seeks results not excuses.

It is wet outside, so I need to put on good rain gear. It is late, but I could get in at least twenty minutes exercise. I want to see that programme on TV, so I will record it and watch it after my exercise. *I am going for results not excuses.*

Now compare open thinking to closed thinking below.

Closed thinking or judgmental thinking. This is good for safety in situations where there could be injury, psychological trauma or death. Closed thinking has recognisable characteristics.

1.   Closed thinking allows only one or two choices, often expressed in the form of a command.

I would like something sweet but I cannot have any because I am fat. *Black and white thinking I have it or I do not have it no compromise, very limiting.*

2.   Closed thinking limits information and intelligence.

I forgot to go for my walk because I am a lazy good-for-nothing. It's no use—I cannot do this; I give up. *No options are put in place, if I fail, I do not learn.*

110

3. Closed thinking is based on punishment—win or lose.

I bolted my food again; I am not doing well; I should be chewing constantly. I am going to exercise hard for two hours for being bad. *If I fail even a small bit I lose and should be punished.*

4. Closed thinking is based on blame and seeing ourselves as victims.

I ate lunch with my friend. I would have chewed but she was eating fast, so I had to as well. Why does everything go against me? It is all her fault. *I blame time, friends, food and other things for my shortcomings, rather than take responsibility.*

5. Closed thinking is full of excuses and failures.

It is too wet to go walking; I will do it some other day. It's too late; I don't feel like it. I will watch TV instead. I might miss something if I go; it's too dark and so on . . . *I have plenty of excuses but little results.*

We need to make sure we understand the critical difference between closed thinking and open thinking. Closed thinking, outside safety situations, leads to a negative, dead-end street and ultimately failure; open thinking develops the mind into a success-oriented positive achiever. Like all the techniques of the sensual slimming strategy, open thinking leads to happiness; open thinking is what happy, successful people do. Happy, successful people use closed thinking, too, but only in safety situations.

2. The language behind a positive attitude. What words to use and how to use them.

The following sentences are affirmations you can use to your benefit. Repeat these affirmations three times a day and, within a few days, they should take effect. They are not directly about being slim—they are about quality of life. Increasing quality of life has the effect of shedding excess weight; trying to shed excess weight while thinking negatively usually does not increase quality of life, nor does it decrease the waistline.

WORTH REPEATING

Increasing our quality of life has the effect of shedding excess weight; trying to shed excess weight while thinking negatively usually does not increase quality of life nor does it decrease the waistline.

An affirmation is a message to oneself that states or affirms something; usually it is followed by action. If I run out of milk for my coffee and say to myself "I must go to the shop and buy some milk", that is an affirmation followed by the action of going to the shop. All our self talk are affirmations. In order to increase the power of your self talk use affirmations with the following rules that compliment the unconscious mind:

1.   In the positive. It's not effective to say "I no longer eat my food too fast", because this programmes in eating too fast. It is more effective to say "I now chew my food thoroughly, enjoying the tastes and textures."

2.   In the here and now, preferably using "*ing*" words. This emphasizes ongoing action in the present. It is not so effective to say "I now enjoy exercise"; this is more a statement. It is more effective to say "I am now enjoying exercise, more and more"; this implies a process, a "doing it now".

3.   With no absolutes, such as *always* or *every time*, which might not be realistic. It is not effective to say "I always chew my food forty times a mouthful every time I eat"—this is not realistic. We may be eating a tough steak or yoghurt that requires more or less chewing. It is better to say "I enjoy chewing my food thoroughly and,

112

feeling satisfied, I leave the rest behind." This affirmation covers many options.

4. Use positive emotion. When saying positive things to your self use a powerful positive emotion this will bring about the affirmation much more quickly. Have a strong positive feeling that what you are saying is coming about right now.

Here are some affirmations for improving attitude; you can make your own as well: Just follow the guidelines above.

SELF-ACCEPTANCE AFFIRMATIONS

I am feeling better and better about my body; I know it reacts joyously to eating naturally, exercising regularly, becoming slimmer and lighter, the more I enjoy my life.

I am accepting my body as I am; I am a more capable and worthwhile person.

Life is good because I have choice; I am now choosing to love myself as I am.

I am now choosing a better quality of life, enjoying food, exercise and positive expectancy.

I have always done the best I could with what I had; I am now choosing to think well of myself; I am my best friend.

Use imagination. Use your imagination in visualising outcomes that you want to happen; use all your senses. This shows your brain where to go and what to do. It increases motivation and reminds us to work the programme. When we use emotion along with imagination, this has the effect of powering us toward the goal. Imagination is used with affirmations, and affirmations are used with imagination, one triggering the other. If we use imagination and affirmations powered by emotion, this is an incredibly potent magic.

3. The imagery behind a positive attitude. What pictures to use and how to use them.

When installing a behaviour, you want to see yourself doing and enjoying that behaviour. Make the picture large, bright and close if that feels even better. Lift it up, down or to either side—whatever feels good—and don't forget to use all your senses:

1.   Visual (seeing)

See yourself being positive, liking your body as it is now, doing the things you have been putting off until you were slim enough. See yourself standing, sitting and walking with an upright open posture— no longer hiding your body away, but looking present and joyous.

2.   Auditory (hearing)

Hear people comment on how positive and bright you are; hear laughter and fun. Hear your own positive internal dialogue.

3.   Kinaesthetic (feeling)

Feel the freedom from worry; imagine the feeling of a lighter mind-set. A positive attitude brings a positive posture; imagine feeling yourself standing, walking and sitting tall. Imagine the feeling of satisfaction in your stomach after you have eaten just enough.

4.   Gustatory (taste)

Imagine the taste of your favourite foods and the satisfying taste of fresher, more natural foods that make your body happy. Imagine your taste-buds letting you know when you have had enough.

5.   Olfactory (smell)

Imagine the smells associated with your change in attitude:

expensive perfume or aftershave (because you're worth it); the smell of new clothes; the variety of aromas from good, fresh natural foods. Places you may go to now with your more positive attitude will have new, pleasurable smells associated with them.

Focus on this imagery often, at least once a day. Treat it as inevitable (because it is), but do not make it conditional. Do not grasp at it like it must happen. Imagine it and then let it go; have the attitude that it is happening right now. Combine your imagery, your affirmations and your emotions—and drive them in the direction you want. That is the secret of success.

POSITIVE ATTITUDE USING SYNAESTHETIC VISUALIZATIONS

Visual (seeing). See yourself as a positive, joyful human being.

Auditory (hearing). Hear the sound of your voice, confident and outgoing. Hear others compliment you on your new positive attitude.

Kinaesthetic (feeling). Feel the feelings of being in the now, increasing quality of life.

Gustatory (taste). Imagine food is now a pleasure; you enjoy the subtle tastes of good food.

Olfactory (smell). Imagine the fragrance of good, fresh, natural foods, imagine enjoying the aroma of your meal before you start to eat, just as a wine connoisseur takes in the scent before drinking.

---

4. The feelings behind a positive attitude. What feelings to use and how to use them.

Feelings are the power behind thought and imagery. Without feelings life is nothing. We know how to live through our feelings not through our rational thinking. Feelings are an advanced intelligence the guides of true masters. If we want motivation we know we have it when we feel a compulsion to want to do something. Our thinking words and imagery and body posture elicit feelings. It is not effective to use affirmations and open thinking and imagery without feelings, as feelings are the fuel driving the engines of desire.

WORTH REPEATING.

It is not effective to use affirmations and open thinking and imagery without feelings, as feelings are the fuel driving the engines of desire.

When using your open thinking, affirmations and positive pictures be sure to include positive feelings. Feelings drive the words and pictures deeper into the brain so that the new behaviour can come about faster and more effectively. How to elicit feelings. Think of a time when you were feeling the feelings you want, go back into the memory, see what you were seeing, hear what you were hearing, think what you were thinking and the feelings will be there. When you are feeling the feelings then do your affirmations, thinking and imagery. An important detail is to get into the body posture of that feeling. Posture is important, with each position or posture there is usually a corresponding feeling. In general we have a stooped heavy posture when we are feeling bad and an upright light posture when we are feeling good. Find out how you breath, how you hold your head up and what expression is on your face. Use your body posture to get the feelings you want for your positive programming. Have a

Web: www.mulrannyparkhotel.ie
Mulranny, Westport, Co. Mayo
Tel: +353 98 36000 | Fax: +353 98 36899
Email: info@mulrannyparkhotel.ie

MULRANNY PARK Hotel

091 - 556777

239 1057

087 - 480

16.06
15.45
15.16

16.05
15.66
15.46

15.30
15.00
14.41

general feeling of already having achieved your quality of life, this will speed up the process.

Rational, positive thinking with emotion is an effective way of leading life; it is a duty of all humankind to think well. What we think about comes about. If we think about ourselves being fat, then so be it. If we think about ourselves struggling with food, then so be it. If we think about ourselves as slim and enjoying life, so be it. The conscious mind makes the target and the unconscious mind follows it.

Sometimes we say to ourselves that it would be wonderful to be slimmer and then we make an image of being fat in our minds. This type of thinking causes us to be fat; imagery is generally more powerful than words. If we are wondering how we failed to become slim, all we need to do is remember the thoughts we were thinking about ourselves and our bodies. Every thought, word or image that we think in our minds programmes our minds. When we imagine ourselves chewing and enjoying our food, going for our exercise, and using open thinking, feeling good, we are programming our minds accordingly.

The other drawback, of course, to negative self-talk, or negative imagery, is that it destroys motivation. In fact, there is absolutely no reason to think negatively at all, except in situations where safety is a concern but, even in these situations, too much negativity can compromise us if we are not careful. We would be better off completely discarding thought patterns of negativity and gradually replacing them with positive, helpful ones. Think negative—be negative; think positive—be positive. The choice, as usual, is yours. *So start now.*

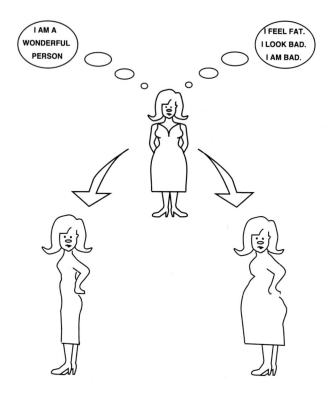

What we think about and imagine, comes about.

Our inner minds can't tell the difference between reality and fantasy when we think with emotion, imagery and detail. When we make images in our minds, then the unconscious mind will lead us towards them. If we think of ourselves getting slimmer, then the unconscious mind figures out ways of getting our goal. When we think of ourselves as fat, the unconscious mind has a difficult time moving towards being slim, because the target it has is fat.

Make an image or images of yourself being happy and doing what you like doing. Better still, fantasise the whole process. See yourself chewing food thoroughly, leaving some behind on your plate and feeling satisfied. See yourself going out and doing exercise, enjoying the good feelings of movement. See yourself now as a more positive, more joyous person. As you are visualising, or making images, you are programming the mind, essentially giving it the addresses towards which you want to go.

WORTH REPEATING

Our inner minds can't tell the difference between reality and fantasy when we think with emotion, imagery and detail. The mind will go towards what we picture and say to ourselves.

Because of this, whatever we picture comes about, including even the things that we don't want.

CASE HISTORY

A client came to me to lose weight, he had heard my reputation and had travelled a long way. He explained that he could only see me once every month. After the first session he came back with little or no change. He said it was great for a while and then as the weeks wore on he lost motivation. So we worked on his programming techniques. We made out affirmations and visualisations that he liked. We ran through all his negative thinking, identified where he was using closed thinking and turned it around to more open thinking. We used the feelings he recalled from having passed his driving test and linked them with his posture which he used during his affirmations and visualisations.

After two weeks I rang him to find out how he was getting on. He reported that after the second session he did well for a few days and then started to go back to his old habits. He forgot to do his programming. I pointed out that he needed to install a reminder to use the programming. It is not that we lack the will to do something, it is often we forget to remind ourselves to do it. It is also better to have the reminder set in as part of the routine of the day. After another week I rang him again. He found that if he used a ritual before he ate to remind himself to chew and enjoy his food that was more successful.

He said a kind of grace before meals prayer that included gratitude for the food and a reminder to chew. His attitude was getting more positive and his exercise started to increase.

He made this happen by visualising himself exercising with a big smile on his face. Sometimes he would feel disheartened as he looked at himself in the mirror before he broke out of the judgemental closed thinking. I advised him also to be grateful for the body he has now and focus more on increasing quality of life not on getting slim. I also asked him to act as if he had it now, a positive mindset enjoying food and enjoying body movement.

The next week I rang him he reported that having the feeling that he had everything now increased his motivation. He began to act as if he had everything and exercise more, enjoy food and feel good. He began to use open thinking in his work and relationships and it worked very well. He reported that after a while the chewing became automatic and the routine of positive open thinking was automated as well. He was now engaging in more challenging exercise and felt youthful and strong again and of course he was becoming lighter.

A more direct route to happiness

There is a kind of conditional series of steps we use to live life and, sometimes, we get them the wrong way round. We do things, to have things, to be happy. We work to get money, to buy things to have, to be happy. Sometimes we forget the happy part, because we are so busy doing and having. Sometimes, before we get to happiness, we die. We waste all that time trying, doing and having instead of being. If we were paying attention to the little things that bring happiness, life would be worth it. It is much better to live unconditionally; we deserve happiness. Be happy, do your work and have what you want.

In an unsuccessful slimming strategy, the steps to the outcome are sometimes back to front and, often, that is why they do not work. Consider the following:

I am going to diet and exercise so that ==== I become slim so that ==== I increase quality of life and do things I enjoy so that ==== I'll be happy.

In this case, happiness is postponed until the end of the line, which is, in a lot of cases, a long way off. A much more satisfying process is to begin to choose happiness now and, as you know, we can get a lot of happiness out of eating and enjoying food and exercise. A successful eating strategy is like this:

Increase quality of life; do things that I enjoy ==== experience happiness ==== become slim.

Experiencing happiness now allows us to choose slimming activities because they are fun, not because we "have to" do them. Happiness now is not going to wipe out our motivation to be slim—it's going to enhance it naturally. This produces better self-acceptance, which produces more motivation.

Conclusion

Attitude is important. A positive, rational attitude brings us success; a negative attitude does not. Unite the mind and body into one powerful force by unconditional acceptance; focus positive thought and imagery to lead to happiness and contentment. Develop the habit of a positive attitude; it may take time, but you're worth it. Keep practising till you have mastered as many happy habits as you can. Use your words, feelings, pictures and posture to develop positive behaviours of happiness. Set reminders, put it into a routine and practice often. (*See The Sensual Slimmer Work Book* for more details.)

Chapter 9

The Happy Habit of Enjoying Food

Eat the way we are designed to eat—
to increase quality of life and happiness.

Chapter overview

We are omnivores, not carnivores or herbivores. Our bodies are designed specifically to eat a certain way so that we can allow our natural sensitivity to guide us. Chew your food at least forty times a mouthful. Make friends with food, and enjoy the relationship. Food is meant to be enjoyed. Lots of people say, "But I enjoy food too much." Overeating is not enjoying food; it is abusing it and yourself. Food should bring you satisfaction, not over-fullness and discomfort. Feeling guilty while eating food, or denying food altogether, also has nothing to do with enjoying it. To increase our quality of life, we need to develop the habit of enjoying eating which, along with exercising, happens to be one of the two activities that support slimming.

The power in the process

Let's recap on what you already know. When we grab a bit of food, slam it into the microwave then gobble it down, we often miss the first step in enjoying food—and that is to experience the anticipation of food at meal-times. This is as important a part of eating as enjoying the food itself. We use our sense of smell and our eyes to appreciate the food. This actually starts our digestive system. We begin to salivate and our stomach produces acids in anticipation of the food it's about to receive.

It is important to get into the here and now. It does not take that long to look at our food and anticipate the pleasure we are about to receive. Now is the time to examine the food and maybe taste some of it to see if we would like any additional flavours. So many people pour a huge amount of sauce or salt on the food before they even start. This is a mistake; unless we have cooked the food ourselves, how do we know how it tastes?

The only thing we need to do now is practise chewing our food. Every time we place food into our mouths, we chew it, taste it and enjoy it. That's the deal. It does not matter if the food we are eating is a biscuit, a dinner, a sandwich, a currant or a peanut; the action is taste and chew, chew, chew. Think about liquefying your food: Human beings need to swallow fine soup. Chew thirty to forty times or more for foods like breads and vegetables. Yoghurt and fruits require far less. If we are eating a steak or tough food, then chewing up to fifty times or more may be necessary. This is what our bodies are made for; if we are eating any faster than that, or chewing less, it's a strain on our system. If we are chewing any less than that, we cause all the negative symptoms and strategies to line up and come into our lives. Yes—all we need to do is chew; get this right and, basically, everything else usually follows from it.

A good way to get into the habit of chewing and enjoying our food is to remind ourselves every day. Sometimes I give my clients a set of affirmations to read to themselves every day. The affirmations serve as reminders to enjoy food and break it down properly for the system. We are changing a habit that we have been doing for many years, and sometimes it takes a while to orientate the mind and body to this new way of doing things.

The snowball effect

Acquiring a new, positive habit is like rolling a tiny snowball down a hill—it gets bigger and it gathers increasing momentum. Chewing food to a fine liquid often has the effect of starting everything else:

➢ By chewing our food we taste it more and release the nutrients within it.

➢ Releasing the nutrients increases energy and we start to exercise.

➢ As a result, we become conscious of how much we are eating and then eat less.

➢ We feel better about ourselves as we nurture ourselves naturally.

➢ Obsessive thoughts about food and slimming stop.

➢ Self-esteem rises and we start to enjoy exercising for its own sake.

➢ The first thing we often note is that clothes become looser as we start to get lighter.

➢ Getting lighter is a kind of a side effect of an overall increasing quality of life, which is actually more important.

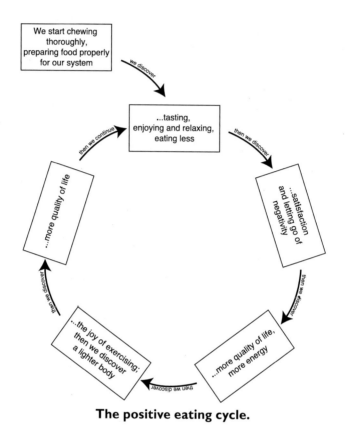

The positive eating cycle.

This is a positive eating strategy. In general, it is what my clients report when they are practising the sensual slimming strategy. One discovery leads to another. They just focus on doing one thing at a time. First, they concentrate on chewing each mouthful up to forty times and tasting the food. Then, usually, they start eating less and feeling the pleasant, satisfied feeling. What is important here is: When the negativity fades away, this allows the letting go of any obsessions about weight. As clients focus more on feelings of satisfaction and comfort, they become more sensitive to good feelings from exercise and relaxation. They start exercising for its own sake, increasing their quality of life. Enjoying food and doing exercise become a way of happiness.

126

Eating with elegance

(i) Chew your food up to forty times a mouthful.

Chewing it less than that is not enough. For hard foods like steak, chew up to fifty times. This is not a lot, given that the human digestive system is designed to swallow fine watery soup-like substances. It is not designed to swallow lumpy, stodgy food. Proper chewing will slow your eating down so that you can enjoy it. It also gives your mouth the chance to monitor the amount of fats, sugars and salts entering your system.

(ii) Put a small amount in your mouth.

It is no use stuffing our mouths with large quantities of food and then chewing it forty times because it will not be broken down enough. We need to place manageable portions of food in our mouths to be masticated correctly.

(iii) Be in the here and now, enjoying eating; it is sound emotional intelligence.

Make eating a value; put in the imagination to enjoy every meal as much as you can. When you sit down for a meal, all you have to do is eat and enjoy your food. It is one of the most simple, yet pleasurable, things we have to do in life. So focus on enjoying the food and the company—good taste and good conversation. Be at peace: Eating is not only physically and psychologically good for us; it is sacred. Most religions have a little prayer they say before or after a meal. This is good sense. Whatever your persuasion, be grateful for the food you are about to eat. A prayer or saying puts us in the now, focuses the mind and prepares the system for digestion.

(iv) Relax, you have time; this could be the most important thing you do in the day for yourself.

It's sad when we hear "I don't have time to eat"—it's like saying "I don't have time to nurture myself." If we do not nurture ourselves, we may become stressed and anxious, and our self-esteem may begin to lower. Life becomes harder to live when we are physically and emotionally undernourished.

(v) Be aware. When the feeling of satisfaction comes—stop.

If we are feeling satisfied and continue eating, then we become too full, and that's discomfort, not satisfaction. It is OK to eat the odd sweet thing so long as we take the time to enjoy it and let our bodies guide us into satisfaction. You know you have had enough of a food when the taste of it diminishes.

Developing the habit of enjoying eating

Let's work on developing the habit of enjoying food. A habit, some would say, takes about three weeks to implement. In my experience, this can vary; most of the time it takes less. The reason is that when my clients find out how easy it is to enjoy food and eat less, the habit becomes a joy. The habit of eating too fast is being replaced by the habit of chewing well and eating more slowly. When we are changing a habit, it is good to remind ourselves of it. It is good to monitor ourselves and watch the changes taking place.

When developing any habit it is normal to start and have a few slip-ups along the way. Most of my clients would slip up sometimes and eat too quickly before catching themselves and slowing down. This is normal, as the habit is not yet being controlled by the unconscious mind. Habits are formed by our first being consciously aware we need to change, then consciously reminding ourselves to develop the habit. Then the habit becomes unconscious, and we do not have to think about it anymore; we automatically do it. Usually, before this last stage, my clients are feeling the benefits. When the habit is really a habit, we do not have to think about it anymore—it just happens.

Habit forming

There are four steps in forming a new, positive habit.

1.   Make the habit a goal.

First we need to want the habit; it needs to be a goal. The habit needs to have a significant amount of desire behind it to make it into a reality. Focus on the benefits of the habit and imagine what life would be like as a result of maintaining the habit. Remember, nothing is difficult; it is just that we have not practised it enough.

2.   Consciously implement the habit.

To consciously implement the habit, we need to practise it often physically and remind ourselves often mentally. We need to do it consciously for a while, and then it will become an unconscious habit. Use the affirmations and synaesthetic visualisations to programme the unconscious to implement the habit. As you say the affirmations, imagine seeing yourself enjoying the food, chewing thoroughly; imagine the tastes and textures; imagine the sound of the food being broken down to a fine liquid.

3.   Factor in failure.

This is where a lot of us fall down. We start our diet and we are doing fine until we eat a biscuit and then we give up in despair: "It's no use", "I have messed up again", and so on. Setbacks are natural and they happen all the time, so factor them in. Expect them—they will happen and they will happen all the time—life is not a straight line.

4.   Unconsciously continue the habit.

We practise driving to learn to do it; at this stage it is very conscious. We focus our minds on exactly what we are doing and nothing else. Then, when we have been driving for a while, it comes to us automatically. We don't have to think every time we change gear or use the indicator; all that is now taken care of by the unconscious.

This is the basic habit-forming process. Do you need to think about tying your shoe-lace? It is automatic; you can do it with your eyes closed. When you were learning, however, it was a different matter; you followed a sequence and thought of every step consciously. We don't forget how to drive the car or tie our shoe-laces; once we have learned, we do such things without thinking. The mind will make almost any repetitive action a habit. Sports professionals, in fact any professionals, try and make what they do successfully into a habit so that they can repeat their success. After a time, we do not need to think about chewing anymore; it becomes an unconscious habit.

WORTH REPEATING

Remember, nothing is difficult; it is just that we have not practised it enough yet.

During the day chew your saliva one hundred times, it has an uplifting affect and you are installing the habit of chewing. It takes a little more than a minute to chew one hundred times and you can do it where ever you are. While chewing practice it at a steady pace, do not rush, you will realise that chewing food forty times or more is actually quite easy. Practicing chewing is very important. When we have a habit of bolting our food for many years this can be a difficult habit to change. Chewing your food thoroughly is perhaps the most difficult of the three habits for some people. So practice, practice, practice the rewards are great indeed.

WORTH REPEATING

During the day chew your saliva one hundred times, it has an uplifting affect and you are installing the habit of chewing.

Below is a set of affirmations and synaesthetic visualisations to help you to develop the habit of chewing and eating your food sensibly. Do the visualisations while saying the affirmations and use positive feelings. It is a good idea to carry the affirmations in your purse; they can be written on a little card of convenient size. Saying the affirmations will install the habit quicker than without them and remind you to chew and enjoy your food more.

The progress sheet that follows the affirmations and visualisations will help you to track your progress at forming the habit as you go along. Use repetition and persistence. The secret of success is persistence. It is not talent, intelligence or opportunity that leads to success; it is persistence.

WORTH REPEATING

The secret of success is persistence. It is not talent, intelligence or opportunity that leads to success; it is persistence.

ENJOYING SLIMMING—AFFIRMATIONS

I now chew more thoroughly; I am eating more slowly, enjoying the tastes and textures, feeling that lovely satisfied feeling; content, leaving the rest behind.

Taking good care of my body and mind, I break down food, being kind to my system.

I am kind to myself and my system; I process my food more finely; my body enjoys the feelings of lightness and energy.

ENJOYING SLIMMING— SYNAESTHETIC VISUALISATIONS

Visual (seeing). See yourself sitting there, relaxed and calm, chewing food.

Auditory (hearing). Hear the sound of the food being liquefied as you prepare it properly for your system.

Kinaesthetic (feeling). Feel the texture of the food in your mouth as you break it down; feel the satisfied feeling of eating just enough.

Gustatory (taste). Imagine enjoying the subtle tastes of good, fresh, natural foods.

Olfactory (smell). Imagine the fragrance of good, fresh, natural foods; imagine enjoying the fragrance of your meal before you start to eat, just as a wine connoisseur savours the aroma of fine wine before tasting it.

You may find it helpful to track your progress on the sheet below. Record the date and whether you have said your affirmations for that day or not. Then, for each meal, record whether you chewed your food thoroughly all the time, mostly, some of the time or none. Continue until you notice the habit is forming. If you forget to chew enough times, that is normal; do not fall into the trap of scolding yourself; just do it right next time and move on. Remember you are practicing your chewing to increase your quality of life not to get slim. Slimming will come as a side effect of increasing your quality of life.

Progress sheet. Date _____

Day 1
Did I do my affirmations & synaesthetic visualisations today?
____yes ___no
Did I chew my food, being kind to my system?

Breakfast	None☐	Some☐	Mostly☐	All the time☐
Between	None☐	Some☐	Mostly☐	All the time☐
Lunch	None☐	Some☐	Mostly☐	All the time.☐
Between	None☐	Some☐	Mostly☐	All the time☐
Dinner	None☐	Some☐	Mostly☐	All the time☐
Supper	None☐	Some☐	Mostly☐	All the time☐

Day 2.
Did I say my affirmations today? ____yes ___no
Did I chew my food, being kind to my system?

Breakfast	None☐	Some☐	Mostly☐	All the time☐
Between	None☐	Some☐	Mostly☐	All the time☐
Lunch	None☐	Some☐	Mostly☐	All the time.☐
Between	None☐	Some☐	Mostly☐	All the time☐
Dinner	None☐	Some☐	Mostly☐	All the time☐
Supper	None☐	Some☐	Mostly☐	All the time☐

Day 3.

Did I say my affirmations today? _____yes ___no

Did I chew my food, being kind to my system?

Breakfast	None☐	Some☐	Mostly☐	All the time☐
Between	None☐	Some☐	Mostly☐	All the time☐
Lunch	None☐	Some☐	Mostly☐	All the time.☐
Between	None☐	Some☐	Mostly☐	All the time☐
Dinner	None☐	Some☐	Mostly☐	All the time☐
Supper	None☐	Some☐	Mostly☐	All the time☐

Day 4.

Did I say my affirmations today? _____yes ___no

Did I chew my food, being kind to my system?

Breakfast	None☐	Some☐	Mostly☐	All the time☐
Between	None☐	Some☐	Mostly☐	All the time☐
Lunch	None☐	Some☐	Mostly☐	All the time.☐
Between	None☐	Some☐	Mostly☐	All the time☐
Dinner	None☐	Some☐	Mostly☐	All the time☐
Supper	None☐	Some☐	Mostly☐	All the time☐

Day 5.

Did I say my affirmations today? _____yes ___no

Did I chew my food, being kind to my system?

Breakfast	None☐	Some☐	Mostly☐	All the time☐
Between	None☐	Some☐	Mostly☐	All the time☐
Lunch	None☐	Some☐	Mostly☐	All the time.☐
Between	None☐	Some☐	Mostly☐	All the time☐
Dinner	None☐	Some☐	Mostly☐	All the time☐
Supper	None☐	Some☐	Mostly☐	All the time☐

Day 6.

Did I say my affirmations today? _____yes ___no

Did I chew my food, being kind to my system?

Breakfast	None☐	Some☐	Mostly☐	All the time☐
Between	None☐	Some☐	Mostly☐	All the time☐
Lunch	None☐	Some☐	Mostly☐	All the time.☐
Between	None☐	Some☐	Mostly☐	All the time☐
Dinner	None☐	Some☐	Mostly☐	All the time☐
Supper	None☐	Some☐	Mostly☐	All the time☐

Conclusion

Food and eating are sacred; they are life giving. You are a sacred being, so treat yourself like one. Focus on increasing the quality of your life, and the life of those around you. Eating food by chewing it thoroughly, and enjoying the tastes and textures, is elegance in itself. I notice that people (regardless of wealth or social status) who are truly sophisticated and elegant eat in this way. They have a strong sense of self and usually a quiet charismatic power about them. I have often wondered: Are they like that because they eat in this way, or do they eat in this because they are like that?

Eat food the way the body is designed to eat; the body will let us know how much it needs. The mechanical breakdown of food in the mouth is the most important part of the digestive process. Enjoy food to increase happiness and contentment. In general, if we chew our food well, we eat more slowly. If we eat more slowly, we enjoy the tastes and textures of the food. If we eat slowly, we allow our taste-buds to monitor the fats, sugars and salt intake. If we enjoy the tastes of food, we enjoy nurturing ourselves, and this increases our self-esteem. This in turn fuels our desire to keep ourselves healthy, so we eat according to the way our bodies and minds are made. We increase our quality of life and treat ourselves and the rest of the world with respect. The world becomes a better place because we are in it. Make it a habit to chew well. (*See The Sensual Slimmer Work Book* for more details.)

Chapter 10

The Happy Habit of Movement

Exercise for good feelings and a clean body—
to increase quality of life and happiness.

Chapter overview

The basic strategy is to learn to enjoy exercise and develop the habit of doing it regularly. Affirmations and visualisations will help you turn strategy into practice.

Enjoy the habit of exercise

To recap what you already know: Our bodies are equipped with amazing ways of enjoyment and pleasure, and it is these amazing ways that increase our quality of life. Eating food produces endorphins, and exercise produces dopamine; both chemicals give us a natural high. Eat to enjoy food; exercise to feel good. Slimming is easily achieved when it becomes a mere side event to increasing the quality of life.

Some people are very athletic. They discover the joy of movement at a young age and they simply thrive on it. There are all sorts of reasons why one child discovers the joy of movement and another child may view movement or sport as an aberration. Anything from bad introductions to lack of opportunity may turn a person off the idea of exercise and movement as being enjoyable. Some people are physically endowed with powerful athletic bodies and some are not; this, however, does not mean that both types cannot enjoy movement and exercise. Athletic people do athletic activities and non-athletic people may choose exercise or play that is less athletic.

Exercise can be boring, or seem like a chore, if we do not find the kind of body movement that suits us. There is something for everybody; the important thing to look for is a way to play. Asking ourselves the question "What exercise causes me to have fun, makes me laugh or engages me in a way that I enjoy myself?" is a good start. Walking can be boring, but walking with music, in a forest, up a hill, by the sea, across a meadow can be more enjoyable. Start with small bits of exercise first then slowly build up; do not exercise to the point of pain or discomfort. Remember, while we can be rational beings, we are also emotional beings. When it comes to exercise, use emotion and feeling as your power to motivate, as well as rationality: The more fun we get out of something, the more we do it.

Develop the habit of exercise

Below is a sample of affirmations and a suggested worksheet. If you are not doing any exercise, or you do it a little less than you would like, you can use the affirmations below to remind yourself. You are creating a habit, and to create a habit, you need persistence and repetition. Say the affirmations to yourself two or three times a day and then begin your exercising.

Seek advice from a professional if you are very out of shape. Otherwise, start small and build up. Even if your first exercise is just for ten minutes, gently bring it up to half an hour or more; do it to enhance your life and lift your self-esteem. One of my clients, who had not many hours in the day between her children and her job, decided to park her car a good way from work. That way, she had a nice walk every morning and evening, and her car parking was cheaper, as she was further from the centre of town.

Use the worksheet to monitor your successes. It is important not to scold yourself if you miss a day. Life happens; get up the next day, exercise and move on. If we scold ourselves too much, we create negative feelings around exercise and are far less likely to engage in it. Remember, exercise to:

1. feel good;
2. increase intelligence;
3. clean the body;
4. promote health and happiness;
5. enjoy social interaction;
6. take a break from other activities;

Affirmations and visualisations for movement and exercise

THE JOY OF MOVEMENT—AFFIRMATIONS

I enjoy moving my body, expressing my joy and aliveness, my ability to move.

Movement gives me good feelings and good feelings give me movement.

My body is becoming strong, fit and upright; I stand tall on the earth; I empower myself with my body.

Moving my body increases my quality of life, and I discover new ways to move it joyously.

My body is my best friend; I bring myself joy through moving, cleaning through breathing and caring for my system.

THE JOY OF MOVEMENT—
SYNAESTHETIC VISUALISATIONS

Visual (seeing). See yourself doing your favourite exercise and enjoying the movement and freedom.

Auditory (hearing). Hear the sounds of the environment you are moving in, or the music you are listening to, while you exercise.

Kinaesthetic (feeling). Feel the feelings of your body getting fitter and fitter, and your lungs cleaning out your system.

Gustatory (taste). Imagine the taste of the fresh air while you walk and exercise.

Olfactory (smell). Imagine the fragrance of your environment where you are exercising.

Use the worksheet below to track your success and to remind yourself how well you are doing.

Day 1.
Affirmations and synaesthetic visualisations: yes ___ no ___

Exercise today: yes __no__ For how long? _____
How did I feel before? _____
How did I feel after? _____
What improvements did I notice? _____

_____

Day 2.
Affirmations and synaesthetic visualisations: yes ___ no ___

Exercise today: yes __no__ For how long? _____
How did I feel before? _____
How did I feel after? _____
What improvements did I notice? _____

_____

Day 3.
Affirmations and synaesthetic visualisations: yes ___ no ___

Exercise today: yes __no__ For how long? _____
How did I feel before? _____
How did I feel after? _____
What improvements did I notice? _____

_____

Day 4.
Affirmations and synaesthetic visualisations: yes ___ no ___

Exercise today: yes __no__ For how long? _____
How did I feel before? _____
How did I feel after? _____
What improvements did I notice? _____

_____

Day 5.
Affirmations and synaesthetic visualisations: yes ___ no ___

Exercise today: yes __no__ For how long? _____
How did I feel before? _____
How did I feel after? _____
What improvements did I notice? _____

_____

Day 6.
Affirmations and synaesthetic visualisations: yes ___ no ___

Exercise today: yes __no__ For how long? _____
How did I feel before? _____
How did I feel after? _____
What improvements did I notice? _____

_____

Day 7.
Affirmations and synaesthetic visualisations: yes ___ no ___

Exercise today: yes __no__ For how long? _____
How did I feel before? _____
How did I feel after? _____
What improvements did I notice? _____

_____

Conclusion

Exercise for fun, to clean the body, feel good and increase intelligence. Focus your mind on increasing your quality of life; let slimming become a side effect of your happiness and contentment. If we exercise all of our lives, it becomes easier, because it makes us stronger—mentally, physically and emotionally. What a great gift the human body is; it works simply and yet it is very complex. Exercise is play, a creative movement of the body. Play is a sign of human intelligence and, in turn, creates intelligence. (*See The Sensual Slimmer Work Book* for more details.)

Chapter 11

Results versus Excuses: How to succeed for good

You were born to be happy. Discover the lasting pleasures of positive attitude, effective eating and joyous movement.

Chapter overview

To increase happiness, self-esteem and quality of life, it is important to commit to the three happy habits of sensual slimming: maintaining a positive attitude, eating effectively and engaging in movement. At the same time, be aware of the common excuses and pitfalls that threaten your success. When you rise to the challenge of changing, you will be amazed at how naturally you attain the results you desire.

Commitment and Persistence

We have looked at the ways to best motivate ourselves using positive language and imagery and cutting out negative conditional acceptance. Like achieving any goal, keeping ourselves on track with sensual slimming takes commitment. Happiness and unconditional love take commitment just the same as getting up in the morning takes commitment. If we are not committed to opening our eyes and getting out of bed, then we don't get up. It is therefore important to commit to a positive attitude, an effective eating strategy and some joyous body movement. These are basic, powerful habits that increase happiness, self-esteem and quality of life—and they are free.

WORTH REPEATING

It is important to commit to a positive attitude, an effective eating strategy and some joyous body movement. These are basic, powerful habits that increase happiness, self-esteem and quality of life— and they are free.

In order to effectively attain our goals, we need to find out the difference between when we are making excuses to ourselves and when we are getting results. Excuses are ways that we think up to achieve nothing; we make them seem logical but they are just excuses. When we don't achieve something, we usually have an excuse about why we did not succeed.

For example, if I say I did not exercise today because I was too tired, that is an excuse or a reason why I did not exercise. The result, however, is no exercise regardless of the excuse. What I want to do is exercise often; what I am doing is not exercising—that is the bottom line. I am not doing what I set out to do. After a while, I forget all about exercise and return to my wanting and not having existence.

So what is an excuse and what is a "real reason"? Is a real reason something like "Well, I could not exercise because my leg is in a cast"? The question to ask here is this: "Is there any way I could exercise even if my leg is in a cast?" And one possible answer is: "Yes, there is—I can work out with light weights; I can do literally hundreds of different floor exercises to keep fit." Therefore, "I cannot exercise because my leg is in a cast" is an excuse. If my doctor tells me I must not exercise because my leg is in a cast, and could be damaged by the slightest movement, that is a "real reason", because it is a safety issue. Anything that is really dangerous to health of self or others is a "real reason".

The difference between when we are successful and when we are not is often a matter of using excuses or reasons why not to do something. There will always be challenges in everything we do. Expect them; they are part of the course of life. Think of all the challenges we face every day:

Finding a parking spot
Having a disagreement with a loved one
Waiting in a queue
Not finding something
Being uncomfortable
Feeling sad
Things not going your way
Things breaking down or not functioning the way we want them to
Being upset because we have not done something we were supposed to do
Being upset because other people did not do what they were supposed to do
Waiting in traffic

Challenges are always there; they never go away, and some days there seem to be more challenges than on other days. When you commit to changing your attitude to a more positive, effective one, you will be challenged. When you commit to chewing your food and eating the way your body is designed to eat, you will be challenged. When you commit to moving your body joyously, you will be challenged. The minute you make a commitment to do something, you will be challenged. Things will go your way and sometimes they won't; that's the reality of life—expect it and be prepared.

Why even try to feel better, chew our food and exercise if we are going to be challenged? Because we are going to be challenged anyway, so we might as well get the most out of it by choosing the results we want. Without challenge there can be no happiness. For example, I come home and I am tired so I say to myself: "I am too tired to exercise." It is an excuse because, even though I am tired, I can still exercise. (If I ran home from work doing a mini-marathon, then I could say I am too tired to exercise—but then again, I would have already done it).

WORTH REPEATING

Why even try to feel better, chew our food and exercise if we are going to be challenged? Because we are going to be challenged anyway, so we might as well get the most out of it by choosing the results we want. Without challenge there can be no happiness.

So here I am on the couch, not exercising like I wanted to because I am too tired. Later I go to bed, feeling tired. I do not have many feel-good chemicals in my system, as I would have had if I'd exercised. Next day I get up not feeling the best and also not having done what I wanted to do the night before—both of which now start to nag at me and challenge my day. To try to feel good, I overeat and, because I have fallen out with myself, I eat carelessly. I feel out of alignment with myself; life is now a little harder for me. I can decide to exercise later and get on with my day and that's fine.

Now if I go home and skip my exercise again, I am even more out of alignment with myself and feel even more challenged. This pervades my entire mind-set and I get even more upset, putting off exercising longer and longer. This sets me up for negative internal dialogue, which then crashes motivation, and back I go to the couch, the TV and to stuffing in food. I now feel bad about myself, and everything I do becomes a challenge. There is no escape. So we might as well go and enjoy exercise, because it is actually the easier option. The habits of exercise, maintaining a positive attitude and eating elegantly are the easy options, much easier than not doing them and feeling bad.

CASE HISTORY

A client who was overweight came in to see me. It was his third session, and he told me that he had not gone out for his walks because of the weather. It was a wet week and he would have gotten wet and might have caught a cold if he had done his exercise. I said this is the west of Ireland; you have lived here all your life; if you expect to walk only when it's dry, you are in the wrong country for achieving your goal. I looked at him squarely in the eyes and said that was an excuse. He looked away and said, "Yes, you are right. I suppose I could have put on waterproofs and warm clothes and gone out anyway."

"So what kind of weather needs to be out there in order for you not to do your exercise and still be true to your commitment?" I asked. "A hurricane," he replied, "but even in a hurricane I could find a safe place to stay indoors and do floor exercises."

He went on to tell me that he had felt worse and worse as the week wore on, until he felt so negative he wanted to give up, because he was failing yet again. What he was experiencing was the challenge of not being challenged, which is always far worse than the challenge. He said he "had no discipline".

I explained that discipline is co-operation with the self, not something that is imposed by an outside force. His next session was much more productive. He had been out for his walk every day since the last session, even though the weather was worse. He reported feeling much, much better, and for the first time in his life, he was enjoying meeting a challenge. It was something he thought he could never do, but when he realised that running away from not being challenged felt a lot worse than the original challenge, he suddenly found his discipline.

"I always hated making myself do something, but then I realised that I was doing it for me anyway—it was a challenge I made for myself," he said. And he was surprised at how much freedom and joy there was in a little discipline. When he compared the constant dissatisfaction of not doing, to the satisfaction of doing, it would not matter if there were a torrential rain—he would still go out. Why is it that discipline can be freeing and even joyful? Because discipline is co-operation with the self. When we are not co-operating with ourselves in the right direction, we do not tend to feel good. Do you feel good in a work or personal relationship when the other person is not co-operating with you? No. Do you feel good when you are not co-operating with yourself inside? No.

WORTH REPEATING

Discipline is co-operation with the self. When we are not co-operating with ourselves in the right direction we do not tend to feel good.

The Most Common Excuses

Now I will share with you the excuses we use to try to smoke-screen ourselves into not doing the programme. You may add any that you can think of, but remember they are just excuses. The way to see through excuses is to put them to honest questioning. Use open thinking skills. Excuses are what we think up to try and fool ourselves into failing. Pitfalls are attitudes or ideas that lead to an ineffective strategy. Let's do a checklist of the excuses and then move on the pitfalls; it's good to get both out of the way.

Excuse 1. This excuse is one of the most common: "I did not have the time."

What we are really saying. " My priorities are messed up; my health and happiness are low values."

If you don't have time to support your health, you have a time-management problem.

A natural-eating strategy is part of what we need to do all day, not something outside of our day.

What to do. Make it a point to chew thoroughly everything that is put in your mouth; it is the way our bodies are designed. Make time.

How to do it. Be consciously aware of your goal when eating; only swallow liquid food.

Excuse 2. "I forgot about it."

What we are really saying. "I did not remind myself."

What to do. See the affirmations in the previous chapter and say them regularly.

How to do it. Put the affirmations beside your bed. Say them first thing in the morning and again at night. Carry your affirmations around with you and say them before each meal. When natural eating becomes a habit, you don't have to say them anymore.

Excuse 3. " I was with so and so, and I could not very well chew my food properly because they were not doing it." Or "I was feeding the kids and so was snacking; I could not do it."

What we are really saying. "The person I was dining with was wolfing their food, so I decided to do the same and mess up my health as well."

What to do. Chewing food thoroughly is a very healthy process for the body and the mind; show others by example; you are enhancing their lives.

How to do it. Tell your friends what you are doing; they will thank you for it. Slowing our eating is a very relaxing way to unwind and is a very good way to be in company.

Excuse 4. "It is too much trouble."

What we are really saying. "I am afraid this will work; then I will have no more excuses to feel bad."

Break the cycle now—you are worth far more than this.

What to do. Realise you are creating a habit. It takes a bit of self-reminding for a couple of weeks and then it becomes something that is automatic; we do not have to think about it anymore.

How to do it. Be in the now. If we feel "its too much trouble", we are obviously not in the here and now while we are eating.

Excuse 5. "It's too slow."

What we are really saying. "I'm still wolfing down my food."

If we find chewing our food thoroughly too slow, it means we are eating too fast. Do you want to go back to dieting . . . stopping . . . putting on more weight . . . dieting . . . stopping . . . putting on even more weight . . . and so on . . .?

My clients report that while they are taking longer to eat smaller amounts of food, the time taken eating is actually sometimes the same. Be patient, in a few weeks time, maybe sooner, you could be shedding weight. Not only that, but you will feel better in yourself. Then, in a few months , depending on how much you want to shed, you will be at your ideal weight, and you will stay there. Oh yes, and your quality of life will be better. You are going to practise this system for the rest of your life, because this is how your body and mind are designed to be.

What to do. Time your meals. How long do you actually take to eat a meal? Remember, along with your meal you may be getting much-needed relaxation.

How to do it. Bear in mind that eating is important; chew thoroughly; it will feel slow if we have been eating too fast.

Excuse 6. "It's too easy." Or: "It's too simple; it could not work."

What we are really saying. "It's too simple; unless I suffer I don't deserve a reward." "How could such a positive way of life bring me such positive results?"

Hundreds of thousands of people reading this book are becoming lighter in mind, body and spirit. This process is a challenge, not a punishment. Your body has all the equipment to enjoy food and to let you know when enough is enough. Just listen to yourself; be good to yourself; eat food the way you are designed to.

What to do. Bring your attitude up to a more positive one.

How to do it. Imagine yourself eating and enjoying the process; use synaesthetic visualisations.

So what is the difficulty in engaging in this natural eating strategy? Getting rid of negative eating habits, such as bolting our food and eating so much we are uncomfortable, is easier than many people think. If we stay focused on chewing our food the way our bodies are designed, this will take from two to three weeks to become a complete habit.

Sticking with it

Natural eating is a slower technique than an all-out starvation diet. Some of my clients can take as little as a few days to get results and others as long as three weeks. In the feel-good department, it is almost instantaneous—it happens now. Remember, it is important to eat naturally for

(i)   emotional well-being;

(ii) mental and physical relaxation;

(iii) social connection;

(iv) proper digestion and elimination of food;

(v)   ingesting the right amount for slimming.

The Most Common Pitfalls

Pitfalls are attitudes that indicate we have not taken on the process completely. A pitfall is usually a sign that we are caught up in old defeatist ways of thinking, and are therefore more likely to fail. A pitfall tells us that we need to focus a little more on the happy habits.

Pitfall No.1

We ask the question "How long will it take until I'm at my ideal slimness?" Good question, but it highlights that we are not focused on our quality of life yet and still too much focused on being slim. A lot of people fall into this one. They go through all the ideas of enjoying food, chewing thoroughly, focusing on quality of life, loving the body, being good to self—and yet they are still in the grip of having to be slim in order to be acceptable. Their focus is still primarily on being slim with all the underlying corruptive conditional conflict. If we eat our dinner while focusing on the dessert, we do not enjoy our dinner. (After you have fully implemented the strategy of sensual slimming, it's usually up to 2 lb / 1 kilo a week, actually).

Pitfall No.2

Some clients give up too early. They can be so entrenched into negative slimming patterns that they try the sensual slimming process for a while and then give up after a few days. They cannot believe that a process of enjoyment and self-approval can work. This process varies from person to person because we are all different. Some people get it straightaway and, within a week, they begin to lighten. Other people can take as long as three weeks, because it takes a while to implement all parts of the process. Once it's in place, that's it, however; people get good results while learning and practising the strategies of positive attitude, chewing and moving.

Pitfall No.3

Some people look at the process as a temporary thing to practise until they have reached their ideal slimness, and then they stop. What happens? Yes, they go back to old, negative habits and put on weight again.

This is for life; this is the way we are designed; this is the way we are: self-respecting, high-esteem-driven omnivores, enjoying the goodness of life in a balanced way.

Pitfall No.4

This is where a lot of people flounder. They refuse to give up their negative attitude towards themselves or towards food. Remember, we must give up all negativity, not just some—all. Let go of negative imagery, the way we talk to ourselves inside, our feeling about ourselves. We need to think well of ourselves, pursue quality of life, and eat the way our bodies were designed to eat. At the same time, it is not necessary to become completely positive in order for the strategy to work. But the more positive we become, the faster it works.

CASE HISTORY

A client came to me and she had to lose a few stone; this time, however, it was doctor's orders. Her doctor had warned her about her weight and recommended that she work with me to reduce it. I introduced the strategy, and she told me that it would not work. I asked her how she knew it would not work and she said, "It is too simple." So I asked her if she had tried the method before and found it wanting. She said she had not and, again, I asked how she knew it would not work.

She said that she had tried every method available to her and none had worked; my method was not going to work either. I then asked why was she here, wasting her money and her time. She said that, well, it might work and she had to try everything. I quizzed her on the other diets she had tried and it turned out that she had never actually stuck to any of them.

I asked her to chew food forty-plus times a mouthful, enjoy food and start her exercise with a short little walk of just a few minutes and then build it up. She agreed and off she went. Her next appointment was what I expected. She did not chew her food because she did not see how that would help and wolfed it down as usual. She did not go for her short walks because she had no time and could not see the point—and anyway, this was not going to work. Then it came out that she'd heard of a surgical technique by which they staple the stomach to make it smaller. Her eyes were firmly fixed on this drastic but convenient technique. "If they staple my stomach, then I can't eat too much, because it won't fit."

> I asked her if she was aware of the long-term
> impact the procedure would have on her digestive
> system, and she replied that it was the only solution
> for her. Then I asked why was she here if surgery was
> the only solution, and she said that her doctor had
> told her that surgery was a last resort; she had to
> prove to her doctor that everything else would fail.
> Essentially, she was coming to me to prove to the
> doctor that she would fail, so that she could get her
> stomach stapled. When this happens to a person, we
> begin to realise that they are on a course to self-
> destruction. It is difficult as a carer to deal with, but
> we must let them go. We can only show people the
> way; we cannot force them.

Change is a human being's most scary word. We work hard at making life into a habit so that we can live comfortably and don't have to think too much. Some people die in their thirties and are buried in their seventies—they make life too predictable and too safe. Happiness has a little to do with challenge and effort, however. We can be very comfortable, and very miserable, if action and challenge are not part of our lives. The trick is to make a habit of challenge, action and comfort, so that they are in balance in our lives. In fact, if there is no action and challenge, comfort does not exist. For example, we want to go for our walk, which is challenge; then we go for our walk, which is action; and then, afterward, we rest, which is comfort. Work, play, rest—in every thing there is the opportunity for challenge, action and comfort. We can also choose not to go for our walk, which is trying to go for comfort but not challenge and action. After a while, we feel stale, fed up; we have none of the mood-lifting chemicals in our bodies that would have been there if we had gone for a walk.

There is no point sitting on the couch wanting to feel good but doing nothing about it. In other words: "I want to be happy, but I do not want to do anything to be happy."

CASE HISTORY

A woman came to see me and we worked together on the system of enjoying food by eating slowly and chewing well. She assured me that she accepted her body and loved it like it is. She was having minimum success with the technique, which was puzzling me at the time. During the second session she mentioned that she did not like being photographed because of the way she looked. I pointed out that not being photographed was a sure sign that she did not accept herself. She insisted that she felt OK about herself and her body. Later in the session, she mentioned that when she had the weight off, then she would finally be happy. Alarm bells went off in my mind.

I again reiterated that the process would not work if she did not let go of the negative feelings towards herself and her body. I showed her how conditional acceptance would not work; she would be de-motivated if she would not allow herself happiness unless, and only unless, she was slim. She did not show for her next appointment and, when I rang, she told me that the process was not working. I explained how the non-acceptance of body and herself will cause the process not to work. She said that she could not believe that accepting herself, as she is now, would make the change. "If I accept my body the way it is now, and if I am happy now, then why would I change?"

"You would change," I said, "because our happiness is not based on a slim body and our motivation is not based on negativity." But she still refused to let go of her negativity. She had tried every diet under the sun and, of course, none of them had worked. Essentially, she was saying "I want to slim, but I do not want to accept myself until I am slim." This is what we call a double bind. To slim, I need to accept myself as I am; then that frees up the motivation to slim. If I cannot accept myself until I am slim, but I cannot slim until I accept myself, I am now caught in a double bind, and I am going nowhere.

Months later she called me up again; she had gone on another diet and failed as usual. She was willing to give it another try. We did a little self-esteem work and again started her on the chewing forty times a mouthful. She agreed to start to let go of the negative attitude towards her weight and her body. She began to notice the feeling of satisfaction and discover the real taste of food. She was slow to get started on her body movement but eventually decided to park a mile from work so that she had to walk at least two miles a day. Then she began to discover that her mood had lifted and she began to feel lighter. It did not take long until she noticed her clothes begin to loosen, and her consumption of food had decreased by a third. She reported that she never would have believed it worked—it seemed too simple and too positive. Change is about challenge, not suffering.

This client felt she had been locked away in a miserable world of self-obsession, always focused on not eating, experiencing guilt feelings when she did eat, dissatisfaction with herself and her body and constant failure. Now she was free. Since then, she has sent me more and more clients. She said that, for her, the best thing about the system was the good feelings about herself—the actual slimming was wonderful but less important.

So now you know about the process. If you have not started it yet, I suggest you do so now. This book will be a great companion for you, and the good news is that the strategy it puts forth is already built into your system: You were born to chew food thoroughly and enjoy it. You were born to be happy; you were born to enjoy body movement. An effective way forward is to make the book a companion for you throughout the process. Reread it as you go through the process to constantly remind yourself of the good you are doing for *you*. Be sensitive to how your feelings and self-concept are improving as you gradually shake off negative criticism, discover the pleasure of food and enjoy body movement.

As you are now practising the process, you can understand how easy and simple it is when you stick to it. One of the things that you may be experiencing now is the ease with which you change. This is a very valuable process to experience as it translates itself to every other part of your life so that you are in constant harmony. Other things that you want to improve in your life become easier. You begin to discover the noble part of you within and the beauty of who you really are. You become an inspiration to all around you. If you are a parent, it is one of the most precious gifts you can give to your children. You know the pain of being obsessed with food and the futile self-absorption, so co-operate with yourself and stop it—now.

Conclusion

Over the years since 1997, I have implemented the sensual slimming strategy with many, many clients—and with great success. My clients represent all walks of life, all ages and backgrounds. Many of the insights in this book emerged because of clients taking on the strategy. Its principles worked for them and will work for you.

We owe it to our bodies and minds to eat sensibly—and sensually. We owe it to our children to teach them the same, giving them quality of life. We owe it to the earth—do we really need to consume so much? The sensual slimming strategy is completely natural, increases your quality of life and is very good for your mental, emotional and physical health. Important message to health professionals- teach them how to eat, most of them already know what to eat.

Enjoy . . .